Healing Sounds for ADHD

Dick de Ruiter and Danny Becher

H*ealing Sounds for*
ADHD

New therapeutic insights

Binkey Kok Publications – Haarlem/The Netherlands

© 2007 Published by Binkey Kok Publications, PO Box 317, 2000 AH Haarlem, The Netherlands (e-mail: post@gottmer.nl) Binkey Kok Publications is an imprint of Uitgeverij Altamira-Becht BV, and part of the Gottmer Publishing Group BV, Haarlem, The Netherlands

Translation: Dick de Ruiter and Valerie Cooper
Cover design and typesetting: Jaap Koning
Cover photo and interior artwork: Binkey Kok
Drawings: Nelleke Dubelaar and Lisa Borstlap
Printing and binding: Bariet, Ruinen

ISBN 978 90 78302 13 1

www.binkey-kok.com
www.altamira-becht.nl
www.diepmagazine.nl

CONTENTS

Isn't it astonishing that most of us are trying so hard to live a rather inconspicuous life, while it actually should be our aim to let our lives be as intense and exceptional as possible?

Do the math yourself. The truth is: Like autistic children, most ADHD children cannotor hardly can—tell lies. The truth, and nothing but the truth, that is what they all wish for. The wishful truth is that they will truly be heard—with our hearts.

Together, we can work it out.

Dick de Ruiter, Spring 2007

1 INTRODUCTION
Concepts

ADHD: a disorder of attention and conduct, with hyperactivity and impulsiveness

---

The diagnoses attention deficit disorder (ADD) and attention deficit hyperactivity disorder (ADHD) have not been in use very long, but they cover a spectrum of psychological difficulties that have been around a long time. Previously, such diseases were termed minimal brain damage (MBD), later—more correctly—modified to minimal brain dysfunction. Approximately ten years ago professionals in the psychiatric community began using "ADHD" as the collective description for a whole range of children's behavior—and adults' as well—that are obviously more serious than stress-related fits of temper or maladjusted, asocial conduct.

The characteristic features of ADHD are trouble concentrating and excessive energy to the point of not being able to sit still. Children who suffer from this will often react by being quick-tempered, impulsive, and thoughtless, causing small accidents such as falling, tripping and bruising themselves. Their behavior is so obvious that people around them find them hard to handle—it's not something you can ignore or pass off as simple childlike exhuberance. Parents, teachers, and attendants will be able to cope awhile, but when it happens all the time, most people find a limit to their patience sooner or later, and problems arise. Some people may express their frustration through an exchange of verbal abuse, others (unfortunately, they themselves learned no other way) may explode with physical violence. There are precious few people who are able to remain understanding and patient. As a result of these reactions, the child will withdraw into its own little world—as we see happen with autistic kids.

If the child exhibits only a lack of attention and concentration, he or she may be diagnosed with attention deficit disorder (ADD)—the child cannot concentrate, his or her attention drifts in all directions. Restlessness and tension are present mainly mentally, but this will have physical repercussions as well.

Although ADHD has been around for many years, it is nowadays considered a typically recent phenomenon, just like excessive stress and autism. In the last few decades autism has increasingly occurred in the U.S. and Europe, not in the least because of our hard-pressed society, with our 24/7 stimuli, additives in our food, and serious air pollution. Currently, almost one in five children has neurological or learning problems. In the U.S. alone, we are talking about at least two million children!

There are two to three times more boys than girls with ADHD; the exact figures are difficult to obtain because in various countries ADHD is not even recognized and treated, although it certainly does exist there. A complicating factor in research is that it is not considered proper or ethical to study and compare large groups of ADHD children, with or without mediation. It is obvious, though, that in the last few years ADHD has occurred much more often than two or three decades ago.[1]

Of course, as an affliction, ADHD does not appear out of the blue. There are many factors involved in the development of ADHD, and if we can recognize the symptoms early on, we can often correct the child's behavior before it becomes worse. In doing so, we may often be able to prevent a lot of sorrow by using a range of methods and ideas we think may work—a combined approach.

Incidentally, in this book we will always speak of working with children, but it will be obvious that adults with ADHD—the "big kids," so to speak—will be able to experience the benevolent effects of this special approach, as well. I will discuss a number of causes of ADHD, but will not go too deep into the matter, due to the scope of this book. In the Recommended Reading on page 107, however, there are a number of excellent books that describe these subjects in detail. You can also find an abundance of information on the internet.

In the closing chapters of this book I will concentrate on sound therapy; an approach that has not had a lot of coverage yet. I will deal with a number of methods with which parents, teachers, and therapists, may be unfamiliar but that may offer a valuable, sometimes even conclusive addition to the already known methods of treatment of psychological coaching and medication. Because ADHD never arises from just one cause, we cannot expect that there will be just one soul-saving treatment. Actually it is the combination of different approaches that will do the trick. Likewise, the method of sound massage, outlined in this book—CD included—will not manage to do the trick by itself, but rather in coherence with other methods and insights it will guide the child toward quieter grounds. As a result, a new balance, quietude, and recovery may be brought to the child's self-regulating system.

So that the flower may flourish harmoniously.

2 SIGNALS
How to Recognize ADHD in Your Child

Therapists and educators use a number of standard characteristic features that are present in a child in order to confirm a disorder as being ADHD. An examining psychiatrist would consider the child's behavior in light of at least six to nine criteria when diagnosing ADHD.

Scientifically as well as socially, the interest in kids with ADD and ADHD is growing. Is there a possible connection between ADHD and new developments in other fields? For instance, what are the consequences for children with divorced or separated parents and their new ways of cohabitation, forcing children to function in two different households? And what are the results of the fact that nowadays children are likely to have their own TV and PC in their room? This was previously unthinkable. These kids are now being exposed to an overload of information and impressions that they have to face and digest. It is not that big a surprise that something goes wrong along the way.

Recognition

ADHD can be recognized from the following conditions:[2]
- The child has a hard time concentrating on one particular task, whether this is at school (learning and listening to the teacher, being alert) or at home (homework, tidying the room, washing up, communicating normally). This goes with hyperactivity (physically and mentally), restlessness, being quick-tempered, with lots of ups and downs and/or withdrawal into his or her own little cocoon.
- The child cannot distinguish the details, but sometimes does not see the bigger picture, either.
- The child is sloppy and shallow, does not finish tasks.
- The child does not listen—at least, it appears that way; often

it turns out the child did hear what has been said. In most cases there is no eye contact at all.

- Conversations consist mostly of no more than a few words; after that, their attention goes elsewhere.
- The previously mentioned exceptional behavior happens in different locations, not only at home.
- The exceptional physical behavior does not fit the actual age of the child, causing an estrangement and repulsion by their peers. This happens more often with somewhat older ADHD kids who behave as younger ones.
- The exceptional mental behavior does not fit the intellectual level of the child. It happens relatively often that ADHD children act at the intellectual level of children some years older.
- The exceptional behavior continues over a period of more than six months.

Of course, ADHD remains a hodgepodge of phenomena that are mutually and intimately related. And of course we should not forget that each child is different. Especially with ADHD children, various other related as well as unrelated ailments occur rather often, making the approach even more complicated. For instance, 30 to 50 percent of ADHD children suffer from dyslexia. And sometimes there will be no other solution but to resort to medication that treats the symptoms, and afterwards go searching for other ways of dealing with the root ailment. Unfortunately it sometimes happens that a child is incorrectly diagnosed with ADHD. That is why it is always advisable to leave the diagnostics to the professionals.

• • •

Denial

For the loving parents it is often impossible to recognize the first disturbing symptoms in their own child. And more often than not, parents' first reaction to a diagnosis of ADD or ADHD is firm denial: "This cannot be happening to my kid. . . What do you mean, ADHD?"

Exceptional behavior does not evolve instantly. Very slowly, mostly unnoticed, the child becomes more restless and passionate, perhaps more to his or herself, which may give rise to a weaker performance at school. Short periods or instances when such behavior occurs will happen occasionally in almost all children. If there is a continuous, outlined pattern, it may be time to organize a meeting with teachers, the family doctor, youth welfare, or therapist(s). Incidentally, ADHD will mostly be observed and recognized by teachers or coaches.

Dutch psychologist Pieter Langedijk describes it in these well-chosen words: "ADHD, how would you like to approach the subject: as a problem, or as a challenge?"[3] Is your child a problem child or is there something you as a parent also need to deal with? It has often been said that your child is a mirror—he or she will react to the energy you radiate! The danger here is that parents possibly will be drawn into a huge guilt complex, which of course is unconstructive, just as denial is not the answer. Incidentally, it is normal for parents to cycle through these phases, to eventually come to the stage of acceptance of the diagnosis, and consequently proceed to action. An attendant aggravating circumstance will be that parents with one (or more!) ADHD child(ren), after a certain period, will be so extremely exhausted and desperate that they will just not have enough energy left to delve into the situation no matter how positive their attitude was at first! Maybe you recognize this.

In the professional realm, there seems to be a change going on as well, and nowadays ADHD is taken more seriously. Parents can find addresses in the back of this book of associations that may offer the parents a guideline, and refer them to experienced aid.

Admission

Once the signals have been recognized, preferably in an early stage of course, the search begins for effective methods that can be used to lead the child. First of all, the problem needs to be admitted—and brought into the open—and next, the child should be analyzed by an expert. Ultimately a plan of attendance must be constructed, together with one or more therapists—a plan that may be acceptable and manageable for both the child and the parents or coaches. In other words, a plan with possibilities for all persons involved. In this scenario, the child goes through a process of growth, as do the adults who are coaching the child. Traditional healthcare, which fortunately today embraces more knowledge about ADHD, and the alternative approaches listed in this book can be perfectly complementary to one another. Alternative healthcare professionals as well are more open to and appreciative of the more conventional ways of treatment. One does not exclude the other; as it would not make sense to belittle somebody else, which does happen all the time. On the contrary, let us join hands—after all, we are dealing with human lives!

Diagnosing ADHD can be done by investigation and examination. Because of the fact that there will always be a number of problems that influence each other, there is not just one simple method of treatment. The investigation is done in various stages that need to be attuned with each other:

- a talk between the parents and the family doctor or therapist;
- contact with the teacher, or the head of the nursery;
- observation of the child at home, in the nursery, at school, and in the street;
- physical and neurological exam;
- orthopedic (skeletal system and associated motor organs) exam;
- motor coordination exam;
- speech exam.

It is important that there be authorities and therapists who are willing to coordinate, collect, and file such investigations, after which a clear plan can be made for effective coaching and treatment. In view of the explosive increase of ADHD, this does not seem to be a superfluous luxury.

Indigo Children—Children of a New Era

Of course it also happens in the ADHD approach that many movements and authors cross the line and resort to the use of vague and hazy language. Still, it is perfectly clear that a certain (not specified) percentage of children born in the last twenty-five years is showing an undeniably different behavior and self-consciousness than the "normal" kids we are used to, so far.

Even down-to-earth scientists like Dr. Judith Spitler McKee acknowledge these shifts. She writes: "Much recognition I experienced while reading and hearing about these new era children. Especially during the past two decades, very sensitive people are being born, often 100 percent paranormally gifted (unjustly diagnosed as ADHD), with many kinds of allergies. They are frequently having problems at school, they do not want—and are not able—to adapt, as over-intuitive individuals. Many HSPs (Highly Sensitive Persons) will fit this image. Here we have sensitive, impressionable, loving people who will be able to help actually design the necessary changes, which we have always been craving for(www.indigochild.com/authors.html)."

Even at a very young age, these kids are showing a kind of "wise" behavior that definitely does not fit their age.

As described by Nancy Ann Tappe in 1980—she came up with the name "Indigo children"— their characteristic features are as follows:[4]

- They feel strongly connected with people, animals, and nature, and are aware of the natural interconnection of everything.
- From the very beginning they show strong intuitive abilities—psychic abilities, some people may say—and they often express themselves in ways that show deep insight, and certainly not fitting their age. This behavior will often come

together with the gift of being able to communicate telepath-
ically with others.

- They may often be vulnerable and sensitive at all levels, resulting in extreme behavior on more than one occasion. They
often feel like nobody understands them, and as a result they
will withdraw, go and watch TV, or play computer games. This
behavior will then be easily subsumed under ADHD, dyslexia,
or something else, while actually these mindful kids, by way
of another association with other children, can revive quickly
and may have a very happy childhood.
- They will have definite problems with absolute authority
without explanation or choice.
- Initially their IQ may seem very low, but it often turns out,
after individual and adjusted tuition, to be very high.
- They will react very sensitively and be allergic to certain kinds
of food, especially sugar and chocolate, and of course all
products containing these. It will often make them aggressive.
The same applies to—in their eyes—meaningless actions
without any creative input.

In 1999 the book *The Indigo Children* by Lee Caroll and Jan Tober
came out, describing the phenomenon in clear and down-to-
earth language, also with indications as to how we may best associate with these children:

- Treat them with respect and acknowledge their role in the
family.
- Assist them in developing a discipline that suits their rhythm.
- Always give them the freedom to choose, of course within
certain (agreed) limits.
- Never lecture them and never ridicule them.
- Always explain why they need to perform certain tasks. They
will only respect parents and caretakers if they realize what is
behind all these tasks, disciplines, and orders.
- Avoid negative criticism. Let them do things without too
much encouragement, let it be more like a matter of course.

- Better associate with them as a partner or friend, instead of imposing. Be open, to a certain extent, to contradiction and comment.
- Do not push them into directions you would like them to go. Usually they know deep down inside already what they would like to be, or what topics they are interested in.

When we look at this list, wouldn't we all like these guidelines to be applied to the care of every child?! It's ur own effort as parents and caregivers, to learn and apply the skills that could create these new possibilities for children. We need to grow more patient and to be more understanding, in order to deal with our heritage in an endlessly loving way!

The ways of treatment for ADHD listed in this book are just a number of possibilities which, in concert, may turn out to be very effective. Some of these are already well-tried and utilized, others are still practically unknown and will need to prove their value. It is a world that is constantly evolving. Hopefully, many persons concerned will profit by these new insights, and eventually they will be embraced by therapists and parents to be applied with success.

3 IN ACCORDANCE
Exchanging Signals, Action, and Reaction

One of the first questions that come to mind in parents, children, and caregivers is: How does ADHD develop in a child? In this chapter you'll learn that the cause is not as easy to pinpoint as it is with factors contributing to a nasty cold. There will always be a number of causes involved, the most important of which I will describe here.

In order to understand how this works, we will use the current behavior of the child as a starting point. Of course it does not make any sense to call any deviant behavior ADHD, and then hope it will soon be better. Every situation is different, every child is different, every human being is different. Still, we can discover similarities, patterns of behavior we will again and again notice in ADHD people. These can be traced back to a number of causes, which do not necessarily occur altogether at the same time—there may even be just a few. It also happens that a therapist does not recognize the described causes as such, because the knowledge of ADHD patterns is still evolving, and not every therapist will yet have all these new facts at his or her disposal.

Most researchers, however, do agree that there never is just one single cause or circumstance responsible for the occurrence of ADHD. Also, one child can never be compared with another in a sense that every child will react differently to outside stimuli, such as food, and everything that should be in the food, and what should not be in there. So the enumeration that follows is likely to be incomplete, and it's equally likely that other causes, which we earlier did not think possible, will come to light. The good news is that with every new discovery there is a new hope for a different approach, for new and sometimes revolutionary, unexpected possibilities.

Environmental Factors

The direct environment plays an important role in the experience of every child. Some of the environmental factors that may contribute to ADHD are stressful situations occurring immediately before and after birth, as well as during the first childhood years; lack of attention and loving touch; and additives and poisonous substances in the environment such as mercury; and air quality.

Disharmony before and after Birth

The first hours, days, and weeks after birth are of immense importance for the further development of the human being. Even before birth, a child is influenced by the loving contact of both father and mother; an exchange of trusting energy; acquaintance in their voices. In this first period in life the very fundaments are laid, for the rest of the child's life.

By providing an energy of harmonious living in the direct environment of the child during this period, it may be possible to mitigate the impact of ADHD. Moreover, this loving and harmonious preparation will also prevent the mother from having postnatal depression. Regrettably, there are also too many factors in life that may cause prenatal disharmony as well. Continuing to work during pregnancy for too long; too little or no support from the partner (or no partner at all); mother's hormonal imbalance caused by a wrong diet; giving birth in a cold impersonal environment (like a hospital with too many bright lights and too loud noises); arguments and stress at home or in the family;—these too may be among the factors lying at the root of ADHD.

First Childhood Years

The newborn and the young child will react very directly to environmental factors such as sounds, colors, and scents. The period just after birth is comparable to a continuous, intense voyage of discovery, which unfortunately will often be disturbed by disharmony in the most general sense: loud sounds or too much noise, a restless atmosphere in the nursery, and loud colors.

Most young children will function a lot better when regularity and structure have been installed in their rhythm of day and night.

Until now we have covered a number of influences that actually are considered as a matter of course in every child's care, because they apply to everyone. The super-sensitive ADHD child will need help dealing with them more urgently. Everyone can understand that these influences are present in a child's life. The topics that we will cover in this section are actually all just a matter of course in child development, and we must not dwell on them unduly. Certainly in many families and educational institutions there is either none or hardly any attention to these factors. That is why we are doing it here!

Lack of Attention and Loving Touch

It is a well-documented fact and understood by everyone that a lack of constructive, positive attention and a loving touch will cause disorders, even physical ones. ADD and ADHD behavior could possibly result as well.

In the Integrated Childs Core method (ICC – explained further in chapter 5) that integrates elements from Chinese medicine with Western methods, much effort lies in bodywork: massage, loving touch, and learning to hug. On the one hand as an expression of being present for the child, and on the other also as a brilliant way to notice and treat signals and symptoms in the child, which otherwise would not come out. Massage can set processes in motion, on the physical as well as on the emotional level, by developing a better body consciousness and awareness of the breath, and it will rebalance the child, while it will invigorate the special bond between parent and child at the same time. A massage will highlight if there are hidden tensions and stiffness in muscles, tissues, and joints, while also diminishing the level of irritation or provocation in the ADHD child. It also stimulates better functioning of almost every body system that is important for good development, such as physical coordination (mainly walking in coherence with seeing), the breath (both consciously and unwittingly), and the creation of speech. The result will be more self-confidence and, accordingly, a better body posture.

Children who have had a lack of physical contact actually become hypersensitive to touch. It goes to show that in the child without contact—apparently because of this lack of physical contact—the behavior resulting in ADHD will be enhanced, eventually. But on the other hand, by restoring and maintaining this physical contact, this negative spiral leading towards ADHD can be broken.

The sooner the parents learn to work with this method, the faster the results will show. With the necessary perseverance and by watching what the child likes, good results have been made, even with children who have been living in their own little secluded world for a very long time.

Incidentally, all the time spent by parents in loving attention with their child(ren), without getting trapped in meaningless fights or discussions is extremely valuable. ADHD behavior can thus be diminished considerably, which makes sense, because the child will realize that being in contact with people in their direct living space may be also pleasant and valuable.

Hypersensitivity to Additives and Poisonous Substances in the Environment

In industrialized areas we are seeing a significantly higher percentage in health problems in general, as well as cases of ADHD. Bad air quality can be involved here, as well as a lack of safe sporting facilities like gymnasiums and playgrounds. There are also various substances being added to our drinking water, such as fluoride in many states in America. As a justification for this, they claim it prevents dental problems, but it has never been demonstrated that this addition has indeed diminished these dental problems! Moreover, the fluoride that is added to the drinking water is actually an industrial waste product. Personally, I would rather not have this in my drinking water! It has been proven that fluoride will make the people more docile and less critical. During the second world war Hitler even had plans to add fluoride to the drinking water.[5] Perhaps there is a hidden agenda after all? In Europe, fluoride has been banned from drinking water, but meanwhile it is an ingredient in almost every toothpaste "recommended by dentists."

Mercury

The story about mercury is way too long to discuss here in detail, but it has been such a sad story that I need to write some lines about it! There are three ways that, even at a very young age, mercury can enter the human body in unacceptable amounts. Mercury is a lethal poison, which can even pass easily through the blood-brain barrier and in doing so can bring serious harm to the brain.[6] The first way is by the well-known vaccinations at a very young age; mercury will often be added to these vaccines. The second is by way of amalgam that is still being used as a dental filling material, although in many European countries it has been banned already, and replaced by composite. And the third way is by way of environmental pollution. Worst causes are the coal-heated power plants, which are vomiting tons of mercury into the atmosphere every year. In the United States alone the amount is already 48 tons a year, but in China it is an incredible 600 tons a year, with a yearly increase of 60 tons! This is hard to imagine, but it is a fact. And this poisonous mercury is spreading around the globe, penetrating everything, in every plant, in every animal—in every human being.[7]

Where there is ADHD, we always need to examine if there is an unacceptable burden of mercury in the body. This examination can be done in every hospital, but also naturopaths can do this, with special equipment. And if indeed the child has high levels of mercury in his or her body, there are protocols for detoxification available at naturopathic centers. It is important that this dangerous toxin be expelled once and for all from the child's fragile body.

Air Quality

From the foregoing it will be obvious that the air quality also plays an important role in the (mal)functioning of people in general, but certainly in the ADHD child. There have been comparative researches in Los Angeles that have demonstrated that children in polluted industrial districts showed a slower development—physically as well as mentally—compared to children living in more rural neighborhoods. Unfortunately, this is not easily changed. Still we must count this as a contributory factor in the whole picture.[8]

Food

As every parent knows, food can present yet another set of considerations and challenges. Everyone is different, and some people are very sensitive to certain foods. In addition to that, handling meals, the accompanying agreements and structured meal times can be contributing factors to ADHD, including: lack of vital substances, minerals, and micronutrients in food; too much refined food and other causes of nutritional deficiencies; and sensitivity to food additives and pesticides.

Handling Meals, Agreements, and Structure

Earlier I mentioned the necessity of structure for the child's development; this also applies to food. Especially for the ADHD child, fixed and steady items in the day are very important. The mealtimes should be at the usual times, on a consistent schedule. If this is not practicable because one or both parents are working, then try at least to be together at one mealtime a day, and to see to it that it is a nutritious and balanced meal. Some families enlist the help of another family member or a friend, or hire a care-giver to help, who will eat with the child or children. Certainly with ADHD kids, eating is not always a carefree happening; it may be very irritating, especially when the children have the urge to move a lot and cannot sit quietly at the table. You have to al-ways perform a balancing act between the discipline of a steady moment for the meal, engaging the child to remain at the table, and a certain kind of freedom if the urge to move really is not re-strainable. This can, by the way, also be introduced as a kind of play, by introducing short moments of movement at set times during the meal. This may be a round of playing tag, or doing a certain body exercise that needs concentration. If this is some-thing you as a parent are not comfortable with, you can try break-ing up the meal into courses and have the child help carry the dishes to and from the table. Or, if the child is more dexterous, you might use smaller glasses that need to be refilled more often, so you can put the child in charge of doing that.

Shopping and cooking together more often also helps, be-cause it involves the child in the process and demonstrates the rewards of a little healthy discipline. And of course it means that the child can count on spending a certain moment of the day with family in a pleasant way. In doing so, when he or she is a lit-tle older, the child may be able to prepare his or her own meals, if need be, and that will in turn enhance self-esteem. Finally, practice shows us that being involved in the preparation of meals also fosters a healthy appetite in the child.

The basic task here is for parents and coaches to initially fa-miliarize themselves with all these issues around meals and food preparation, and secondly put this knowledge daily into practice, as far as this is possible, of course. Creating this one point of sta-bility will go a long toward helping the ADHD child.[9] It may seem as if I am picturing here an idyllic situation, which will not always be feasible. But we can always keep striving for it, always trying to be there for the child, offering good meals prepared with love.

Lack of Vital Substances, Minerals and spore elements

Just as understandable that the lack of a loving touch will eventually lead to a change of behavior is the concept that a lack of vital substances in the daily food will create problems. And not only on a physical level.

Usually it is because of a lack of elementary knowledge about food, and how it needs to be prepared, that this kind of deficiencies occur. Sometimes this is combined with the lack of time or motivation to prepare a good meal, and resorting once more to fast food, prepared frozen foods, or starchy snacks—the quick fix. Compounding this problem is children can be fussy eaters and parents may be too tired to persuade them to eat good food that isn't laden with fat and sugar.

It is not only a matter of what you put on the table, and the size of the meals, but also the manner of cooking that will determine the amount of remaining nutrients. For example, in 100 grams of raw endive there is about 12 milligrams of vitamins; but when an endive has been well cooked there will only be one milligram left of those twelve! That is why it is advisable to always mix some raw vegetables in with other food that the child will like, such as cooked potatoes. Leafy greens are amongst the most nutritious foods. Chard, collards, kale and spinach have all made it into the World's Healthiest Foods list. The easiest way to cook these is to rinse them with cold water, shake off the excess water and cook them to wilt in a steamer. You don't need fancy equipment to steam vegetables. If you have a saucepan with a tightly-fitting cover and an expanding steaming basket (available even in supermarkets), you've got a steamer! Put one inch of water in the saucepan, place the basket inside. Turn the heat on medium when the water in the pan starts to bubble, place your greens inside and in less than 3 minutes you'll have wilted greens. For denser vegetables like broccoli, steam for 5 to 7 minutes or until bright green.

On behalf of parents with children who do not want to eat anything healthy, I offer the following recipe for what I call an "astronaut drink." Mix thoroughly in a blender a fair amount of bean sprouts, alfalfa sprouts, or mixed sprouts (preferably organic) with a cup of water and a splash of any kind of concentrated fruit juice, strain it, and serve. In seconds you have a drink that almost every child will like, containing all the vitamins and other vital nutrients the child needs!

Of course, you can also opt for food supplements, but it needs to be said that really effective supplements are very expensive; the cheaper ones often contain artificial instead of natural stabilized vitamins, which do not or hardly work at all.

Refined Food and Other Causes of Deficiencies

Little by little it has become commonly known that refined foods, from which most important nutrients have been removed (often by using a whole range of weird agents as well), are not very beneficial to your health, to say the least. The most explicit example of this is white bread, to which later, after everything has been refined out of the wheat flour, all kinds of "healthy" extras are being added. People who do not eat anything but refined products will sooner or later show serious deficiencies, causing even more serious disturbances, physically as well as mentally. Another thing to reckon with is the fact that the buffer after which the body will give up is not as high as it used to be 50 years ago. This could also be the result of eating these refined foods, such as white flour and grains, white sugar, and refined salt.

A good example of the impact that a mineral deficiency can have is a lack of zinc. Expectant mothers generally need at least 25 milligrams of zinc every day; still, most pregnant women will get only 15 milligrams or less through food and drink. Not only may this result in spontaneous abortion, but also the child-to-be will have deficiencies no matter what, which may be a basic factor in developing ADHD.

Not only the intake determines the available amount of substances inside the body. There is also the influence of stress and intense physical as well as mental exertion, or the use of certain medicines that account for the assimilation of certain food particles. Ingredient labels listing minimum daily requirements of vitamins and minerals in products, while helpful, are not always valid for everyone. A well-known example is that smokers need a lot more vitamin C than nonsmokers.

There is yet another aspect to this important factor of deficiencies in the food chain, of which most people have been completely ignorant: the fact that during the last fifty years the mineral contents in our food has diminished dramatically. In vegetables, for example, there has been an average decline of 50 percent! Fact: a carrot in 1940 contained an average of twice as much as magnesium, calcium, iron, and copper as the same carrot in 1990. In magnesium there was a decrease of an average 24 percent, in copper this was a heavy 76 percent. The much-consumed potato has lost in this 50-year period 30 percent of magnesium, 35 percent of calcium, 45 percent of iron, and 47 percent of copper. And in 1991 you would need to eat ten tomatoes compared to one in 1940 in order to get the same amount of copper into your body. Also the intake of so-called trace elements and micronutrients such as manganese, selenium, and iodine, has declined considerably.

This means that while we all think that we are getting sufficient daily amounts of vegetables and fruit, there is actually not enough in it to give us what we need. Also the mutual ratio of various minerals is now much less ideal, which in turn negatively influences our body chemistry. A way to address this problem is to buy organically grown products whenever possible. These contain a better balance of nutrients because the focus is placed on naturally improving the soil and growing a healthy plant that can resist disease and pests instead of hitting the crop with chemical fertilizers and pesticides. The more demand we can create for these products the more willingly the larger agricultural companies will engage in organic farming, and the less expensive it will eventually become.

For now the best we can do is supply our children with vitamin and mineral supplements that are easily tolerated and assimilated by the child, and pay attention to how they react.[10]

We can also experiment a little more in healthier ways of food preparation, as this may also help to keep more vital substances in the offered meals.

Additives

The love you put into even a simply–prepared meal can make up for a lot. But there are other additives that are put in our food and drink that can't be washed away with love! ADHD children are especially sensitive to these kinds of additions. A number of these are utterly superfluous, like colorants. Not only can children react to these additives with extraordinary behavior, but their immune system will also be negatively affected. This may cause a certain over-sensitivity to a whole range of infectious diseases.

The fact that government food inspection departments have allowed a number of these substances for use in the food industry does not mean, unfortunately, that these substances are safe. Many times it has been demonstrated that simply excluding foods –with additives from the daily meals, and switching to natural foods, will erase or at least diminish many nasty complaints—including ADHD symptoms.[11]

Incidentally, cleansers, floor-coverings, and cosmetics contain also substances that may cause physical and mental disorders, when there is regular exposure. That is why as parents you also need to check if your child is likely to react to these products (see "Kinesiology – Muscle Testing for Compatibility" on the next page). Health food stores offer a whole range of cleaning products and cosmetics that are not noxious.

Harmful and Beneficial Food and Drink, Effects of Sugar

It's not always easy to tell whether a substance or food will cause a harmful reaction. One food could be easily digested by one person, but cause an allergic reaction in another. Neither can you say that everything that tastes good to a person will also be good to him or her. A big part of the problem is many people have become accustomed to the excessively sweet or salty qualities added to refined and/or prepared foods, and therefore find natural foods too bland.

Kinesiology—Muscle Testing for Compatibility

It might be a good idea to learn how to do the muscle test—an easy way to discover and avoid products to which a child might respond adversely. These tests come from an alternative health practice known as kinesiology, also referred to as "touch for health." There are many therapists (like masseurs, alternative doctors, healers) who can teach you how to do it.

The muscle test can only be done with a neutral face (no smile) and with all fluorescent lights off. Begin with a test to check if the child (or any other test subject) will react well. The child stands facing you, with arms relaxed and feet a bit apart, so he or she may stand steadfast. Now have the child stretch out one arm horizontally, and lay your own hand on that side on the child's wrist. Lay your other hand on the child's other shoulder, as to keep a balance. Instruct the child to say out loud, "My name is (his or her first name). Explain that immediately afterwards, you will try to push the child's arm downward, while the child is to resist your pressure in order to keep his or her arm horizontal (without too much force). Then do the test. With the child's correct answer, you should be able to feel the muscle block, so it will be hard to push the arm down. You should take into account the child's muscular strength; with an adult you will of course need a lot more power! Now ask the child to repeat this once more, but using someone else's name. While testing this wrong answer, you will undeniably feel that the child will not be able to keep his or her arm up; you will easily push through the resistance. You may do some other double-blind tests, where the child "speaks" the test words only mentally, not vocally. You will notice that even then a positive sentence will always test positive, or strong, and a negative, untrue sentence will result in a weak muscle response. Incidentally, the words of the test person should always be affirmative; so a sentence like "My name is not Peter" would not work. Neither would a test with a question, like "Is my name Mary?"; it should always be "My name is Mary."

The testing position is intended to isolate the muscle from the group that it normally works with. Since the muscle is isolated, it is at a disadvantage. Muscles do not normally work singly, so one by itself is not going to be as strong as if it were used in the usual way. For this reason, it is important to test only the first couple of centimeters of the range of the muscle action, applying the pressure gradually and releasing it gradually. With a greater or sudden force even a strong muscle could be overcome, and this is not the point of the test. The muscle will be strong either in the first part of the test, locking in place, or it will give way completely and swing easily through a larger span of the test area. With normal strength, a muscle can be used repeatedly and not fade or tire quickly. If a muscle hurts during the test, stop immediately, wait a few minutes to let it rest, and try again.

After these test questions you can continue with the real job, like an allergy test, or how many drops of a certain medicine will be the most effective, and so on. Have the child hold the food or the medicine or supplement in its right hand against his or her stomach (the place of the solar plexus, in between the sternum and the navel), and perform the test with the child's left arm.

It goes without saying that you first need some experience in order to test well. So try playing around a bit first with testing friends and relatives, before you apply it seriously.

Finally, a word of caution: sometimes someone who is energetically very much out of balance will react just the opposite, strong with a negative statement, and weak with a positive one, or even weak in both positive and negative. Be very careful, stop testing, and leave the case to experienced therapists.

Diet

There are several food products that we know are not suitable for most ADHD children; these are not to be at all, or at least in much smaller amounts. Fortunately, there are many good alternative products.

- Sugar and all products with sugar, such as candy, chocolate, and soft drinks; these are the usual suspects but many brands of peanut butter have sugar, and sugar is sometimes added to tomato-based prepared products like catsup and even some brands of tomato sauce. Also, buyer beware: the so-called unrefined cane sugar is in many cases just refined sugar mixed with some sugar syrup. Only the dark brown, unrefined sugar from health food shops or health food sections in supermarkets will be nutritious.

    Other good alternative sweeteners (always buy these organic!) are: fresh fruit, dried fruit like dates, raisins, or currants, and other dried subtropical fruit such as mango and papaya (always thoroughly washed and soaked overnight), sugar-beet syrup, honey, and maple syrup. Be careful, though; some children do not react well to honey and/or tropical fruit.

- White flour and all products made thereof (often combined with sugar and/or dairy), like white bread and other highly-processed products, the so-called "empty calories." Replace these with whole grain, unrefined, or half refined products.

- Cow's milk and all products made thereof (often combined with sugar), most of all cheese (cheeseburgers, pizzas, and the like). Some children may tolerate yogurt and buttermilk, but always in moderate quantities. Dairy may sometimes, but certainly not always, be replaced with soy products. Many Western people are allergic to dairy, but many to soy products as well! This can all be tested of course. There are many children who by nature already have an aversion to dairy; Older generations of Westerners—especially Americans—were taught that cow's milk is necessary and nutritious, but in the last decades it has been determined that milk is just not that healthy for everyone. Twenty percent of our population cannot even digest the lactose (milk sugar) in dairy products.

Dairy causes mucus that can block the assimilation of minerals and vitamins.[12] Do not worry so much about a lack of protein or calcium, because first, we do not need so much protein, and second, there is enough other foodstuffs containing protein and calcium: legumes (beans) and whole grains for protein, many green vegetables for most of the nutrients, especially calcium in the right proportion to magnesium (milk does not have this ratio) for best absorption. You might give small children extra tablets of calcium from nettle, or nettle herbal tea. Assimilation of calcium will depend also on other factors, like an ideal combination with ripe fruit (vitamin C) or cold-pressed oil (vitamin D). Ask a good nutritionist about the right formula, because there is a lot of calcium on the market that just will not be assimilated into the body.

- Pork and sausage. As a practical matter, it appears that children have a hard time digesting these; it may contain certain negative qualities, causing the child to be more restless. Responsible elements are the purines, poisonous breakdown substances that are abundantly present in this meat.
- Fatty dishes. Children chew very little, and ADHD children chew even less, because they are always in high gear. That is why it is so essential to have a quiet atmosphere at the dinner table—as opposed to sitting in front of the TV with the plate on your lap! Fried products—potato chips, crisps, and other snacks included—also fall in this category. Of course there are also many good fats, such as cold-pressed, unrefined vegetable oils (sunflower, olive, or sesame oils).

  If you do not chew enough, heavy and greasy foods will put a much heavier burden on your liver. This, in turn, generates aggressive behavior, because there is a direct interaction between the liver and aggression. Chinese medicine knew of these interactive energies two centuries before our era; they are described in acupuncture books from that time.
- Icy-cold drinks and foods. You cannot always deny your child this one little ice cream, but it should certainly not become a

habit. During dinner you should never serve ice-cold drinks in the first place, because the cold fluid will cause the stomach to cramp, so for a long while it will not be able to secrete its gastric juices to predigest the food. This causes the consumed food to pass unprepared into the intestinal tube, and the result will be irritation, gas, and poor assimilation of food substances. Carbonated cola (Coke, Pepsi), certainly served cold, is the most dangerous drink ever. Because of the high amounts of sugar (or substitute chemical sweeteners which are worse) and other ingredients like caffeine,, it will provide a very short-lived moment of pep because, but then afterwards comes a crash, which in ADHD children can spiral into a huge depression.

• All extreme flavors in food and drink—very sour, sweet, hot, or salty are best avoided. Just remember the old adage that "You are what you eat." If you put extreme stuff in your body, you can expect some extreme results! And that is certainly not what we are after.

Sugar, the Biggest Sweetness in Our Society

Today, everyone will agree more or less that refined sugar—including all food and drink containing it—is harmful. What most people do not know is the fact that sugar is the very largest addictive product ever, with a global average annual use of 50 to 70 kilos per person. That is why the sugar industry will never disappear. Together with the unrelenting and exponentially growing use of sugar in the last century came the extensive increase of incurable diseases. This is also a common fact, but it will seldom if ever be openly acknowledged. Too many peoples' personal interests are involved, from the consumer who is "hooked" on sugar, to the industrialist processing the sugar cane or beets, to the poor people working the cane plantations, and all the people they support—and that's just the sugar-growing industry.

Yet, by the same token, personally, one individual at a time, we are able to change a lot! We can choose to decrease or even completely refrain from using sugar. And every therapist who works with autistic and ADHD children can confirm that after a radical stop of the use of sugar, the behavior of all children changed for the better.

Here also, the food industry will follow up on this by recommending products containing only half the amount of sugar, or even sugar-free. But in order to get the sweet taste of course the food processors need to add other chemical sweeteners, like aspartame, which has been proven to have a destructive effect in the body—yes, and even may contain a factor in the growth of cancer.[13] So these substitute sweeteners are not an option.

Hyperactive children are especially sensitive to sugar and everything with sugar, for it causes an excessive stimulation of various endocrine glands, which in turn disturbs the creation of certain substances in the brain. This not only stimulates hyperactivity, but also interferes with vitamin and calcium assimilation, resulting in all kinds of bodily imbalance.

So it would pay off, as a parent of an ADHD child, to study this matter, and immediately moderate the child's use of sugar (and of course set an example, yourself). My own experience is that with children it is advisable to very gradually, almost imperceptible, reduce the sugar contents in food and drink, because even in these young children, sugar consumption has become a habit and an addiction. If you were to stop too abruptly, it could easily result in associated side effects, like (more) mood changes, from very active to very apathetic, with fits of crying and even suicidal behavior!); certainly, with ADHD children, we really do not want that!

There are sufficient alternative sweeteners that do not have the devastating effects of sugar, but you need to get to know how to use them in your cooking. You will find these products in health food stores. Choosing brown cane sugar is not really a solution, because it is often as refined as beet sugar. Good products are (in order of sweetness):

- unrefined, dark brown beet or cane sugar (still containing all original nutrients);

- several kinds of honey (neutral taste for in tea, but also very specific kinds like buckwheat honey on toast);
- maple syrup (grade A only); and several kinds of malt syrup (made of barley, wheat, or rice).

For specific occasions you can even use raisins, figs, and/or dates, by slowly cooking them in water for a long time into thick syrup. Again, in most people and also in children, the taste buds are so desensitized by too much sweet stuff, it will take a while to gradually get used to less sugar. Eventually, a tiny bit of honey will be enough, or even not at all needed anymore, for instance in lemonade or herbal tea.

So, in food and drink, sugar is one of the biggest malefactors. But there are more! I already mentioned the additives. Children in general will react strongly to certain dyes and flavor enhancers such as monosodium glutamate, but much more than in the past they will also show allergic reactions to cow's milk and products made thereof, especially cheese. As a parent you should not react too strictly to this and certainly not work with big stop signs, because this will only achieve the opposite. Again, experience is the best teacher: when the child realizes that it will have much less mucus (physical bother), or less depression and feelings of isolation (mental bother), when not eating these products, he or she will be more inclined to refrain from taking them. Of course, as a parent you can draw the child's attention to this connection between its physical condition and consuming unhealthy food. There are naturopaths who can find out, with a sophisticated appliance (Vega-test and the like), to which foods and drinks a child will be hypersensitive, or even allergic. The outcome will often be surprising! In the case of ADHD it is advisable to do such a test, and to adapt the recommended eating habits.

Incidentally, this applies to numerous substances that are nowadays added to our food, in the interest of longer keeping qualities, more color, taste, or aroma, better structure or baking quality, and so on. Let's look further into these substances.

Hypersensitivity to Additives and Poisons in Food and Drink

Exposure (especially prenatal) to certain chemical substances which affect the endocrine glands (e.g. PCBs) can have negative effects to the development of the nervous system and behavior patterns, and may retard the cognitive development.
—*World Health Organization (WHO)*

In my own practice I once treated a woman who suffered for many years from serious migraine headaches. This had caused her to spend at least one third of each month in bed, and even the strongest pills did nothing. While testing her, it turned out that she was using a certain kind of contraceptive that I immediately recognized from earlier similar cases as the malefactor. A hormone pill like that will not only affect the period, but the whole system of interrelated hormone glands as well. After stopping this contraceptive, her migraines were almost immediately a thing of the past.

This example shows us that the intake of chemical substances in our bodies can lead to physical disturbances. This does not only apply to medicines, but also to the additives in the foodstuffs entering our bodies.

The ever-increasing contradictory media coverage about additives in our food and drink is enough to make anyone's head spin. Although there are food inspection departments worldwide that claim these kinds of additives are safe, there are many examples of people whose health problems diminished after changing over to a more natural diet. Some safe additives are still being used after many decades and come from natural sources; others are made in the lab. Still, we can easily state that for the most part these colorants, fragrances, flavor enhancers, and preservatives originally were not present in our food. They actually do not belong there, because they are a threat to our health, no matter what they say; the same applies to hormone preparations used in cattle breeding. About 90 percent of all products offered in the supermarket contain these kinds of additives—moreover, the greater part of these products are completely superfluous in our society! It is simply mind-boggling. Additives just do not belong in our food and drink, period. To me, it seems convincing enough that when children stop eating and drinking these products, there is a noticeable improvement in their behavior.

Lack of Physical Exercise

Over the last few years it has become crystal clear that children are seriously lacking efficient physical exercise. Now, hyperactive children struggle with a surplus of movement, but I am talking here about efficient ways of body training and movement. Everyone knows that daily physical exercise is essential for good functioning of body and mind, but still there are few people who realize that this needs to be very direct, efficient, effective movement. An ideal way of learning efficient body movement along with deep and efficient breathing, is yoga. It would be a good idea to use yoga or equally effective methods to practice daily at school, for a regular amount of exercise—and relaxation! Parts of the CD in this book could go well with this routine. For the most part, yoga is a breathing practice in order to get a better awareness of the body. Breathing is always the basic movement from which a therapeutic practice may work wonders.

Sound Environment

At the end of this chapter we finally arrive at still another—possibly underestimated—phenomenon which may also partly make up for an aggravation of ADHD: sounds from around us.

In many households in our modern society the sound environment is out of tune. Look (listen!) around at your own situation at home or at work: How often is it not so that you hear heavy traffic sounds from the street or in the air, or loud music from a radio or TV? Even healthy people can get thrown out of balance by these sounds; so it is understandable that such loud noise or music will not be beneficial to kids with ADHD. These loud sounds will literally put us out of tune, in our whole system—body and mind.

Very subtle sounds, such as the constant buzzing of a refrigerator, the hum of fluorescent lights, and even inaudible vibrations also resonate throughout the body and with constant, long-term exposure—can have a negative influence.

I can tell you a story about an electrical alarm clock that was producing a constant, almost inaudible buzz; when taken away off of the bed stand, and out of the bedroom, the children did not have nightmares anymore!

How about all these mobile phones and their emissions? Almost every child is walking around with one nowadays. It has been demonstrated that mobile phones are causing disturbances, for instance in the brain and the hormone system.[14] Of all body systems, both the brain and the hormone system happen to be the ones that are closely related to the occurrence of ADHD. You can draw your own conclusions!

Further on in this book I will elaborate on the influence of sound, and the special possibilities to work with harmonizing sounds and music.

Morgellon's Disease

Morgellon's disease has only recently been discovered and described by medical science. Symptoms are: serious skin conditions with a lot of itching and irritation; a feeling like millions of insects are swarming under the skin; serious fatigue, short-term memory failure and other mental functions often described as a fog inside the head. Often the disease comes with other ailments such as irritable bowel syndrome, multiple sclerosis, even pure psychosis.

Morgellon's disease isn't a cause of ADHD, so why do I mention this still rather unknown disease here? Because of the ignorance about this disorder, a completely wrong diagnosis may be made—like ADHD! This serious ailment is a typical example of the new kinds of diseases that have been cropping up at an alarming rate lately, and about which medical science has no clue how to treat.

Although it is hard to diagnose, and the causes are hard to stipulate, there have been good results with alternative treatments, like the ocean minerals (see description in Chapter 5, page 65), which seem to show promising effects.

• • •

Addictions

People with ADHD are showing a number of common qualities that eventually may lead to compulsive behavior and serious addictions. This coincides with the fact that their ability to produce dopamine does not always work as it should. Dopamine is a substance we produce in our brains when we have pleasant feelings. It belongs to the endorphins, which are chemically similar to and work like morphine. When these substances are being released we feel fine, and in this way they work as an inner reward system. They are of vital importance, because this system is directly related to things like eating and making love.

A similar production of dopamine and the occurrence of pleasant feelings can be obtained by the use of alcohol and drugs, and also by any kinds of activity, such as car racing or parachute jumping, that cause the adrenaline level to rise.

Although not many people are addicted this way, it happens a lot more among people with ADHD. As mentioned before, their brains will release smaller amounts of dopamine than others', so they need to go to greater extremes in order to experience the same pleasant feelings as "normal" people. For people with ADHD, life is kind of like being in a coffee bar that serves only caffeine-free coffee. This makes them take greater risks and strive for zealous goals, like the well-known example of Richard Branson, founder of Virgin Records. The seamy side of these in themselves excellent ambitions occurs unfortunately more often in people with ADHD: a leaning toward self destruction by way of gambling, drugs and sex addiction, procrastination and running from responsibilities, creating one crises after another. The only alternative will be this dull, tedious little life without the kicks, which is not tolerable for everyone. So the continuous striving for stimulation and excitement becomes a kind of addiction.

But still, these are extremes. Yes, they are mavericks. But in general, these people with ADD/ADHD are brilliant, energetic, vivacious people, who—just like anyone else—need to find a meaningful way of living their lives, in which they can continuously be active and find their gratification. If they succeed in this, if need be with careful coaching in their school years through vocational training and the like), it may well be possible for them to live creative and sparkling lives. One of the best methods with which this can be very consciously coached and even profited from, is the DaVinci method (read Chapter 5 for a short description). You will find good examples of those successful people in every country, who are often found enjoying the limelight of accomplishment and even fame.

• • •

Mutual exchange of information

Although in this chapter we have been able to line up a series of possible causes of ADHD, it does not mean that our understanding is complete, no more than we can come to a solution just by acknowledging what causes it. But any good information does contribute to gaining more insight and understanding of the child and the way he or she does or does not call attention.

We see many remarkable similarities between an ADHD child and an autistic child, particularly in the reaction of shutting down when over-stimulated and not communicating at all. The difference is that with ADHD the exchange of information is obviously disturbed, like a radio receiver that has not properly been tuned to a channel. In autism, transmitter and receiver will be completely out of line.

Another thing is that the reactions will often be unexpected and not in proportion to the context; for example an aggressive scream out of the blue would be a sign of inability. We just need to persevere, to try and learn—through better understanding and more insight—to deal with this behavior. No matter what, ups and downs: keep trying!

4   TRUST
Mutual and Unconditional

> Since we now have more understanding of the factors that play a part in the development of ADHD, let's look into aspects of the behavior of ADHD children that asks for a special approach. I am talking about behavior we all are familiar with, but which we hardly ever dwell on.

One of the characteristics of ADHD is that it will be hard for the person concerned to enter into a relationship with someone else: parents, friends, partners. Of course, these relating problems originate at a very early stage; probably in the first few months of the child's life. This is why it is so essential in the child's first stagelife, that the parents do their utmost to anchor trust and confidence in the child. Unfortunately, this will often start off in a rough and insensitive way, by cutting the umbilical cord way too early, and immediately taking the baby away from the mother because it apparently needs to be instantly weighed and dressed. When you stop and think about this, it's a wonder where the common sense and feeling went with the people in the hospital—it seems nurses and caretakers are the only ones stemming the tide of impersonalized care. In this stage, the first deep traumas can originate, which later might be enhanced by insensitive or egocentric behavior on the part of parents and companions, causing the child to think: There, you see, you really cannot trust them, ever!

But hey, these disturbances in a relationship do occur, and the consequences are not always foreseeable. Fixed patterns cannot be altered by giving orders, or by giving a pill. It often takes so much time and effort that many a parent eventually will get the feeling that it is a never-ending haul. Still, here too, the only real possibility of change for the better will be to keep on trying, with patience, giving love and attention. Of course, this does not mean that the child can run off free and do whatever he or she wants! An ADHD child especially needs a very transparent struc-ture—one in which he or she feels able to be his or herself, and that she will not be unduly restrained, because for the child this would mean as much as being smothered.

Keep It Real

More than any other child, an ADHD child will be able to fault-lessly see through unreal and insincere matters, and throw a very bright light on them. A good example is the conditional redemp-tion behavior most parents use, i.e. "If you do this, I will give you that." Especially in the first stage of life, the child's character is somehow be cultivated by this ability to see through this kind of manipulation, it is fixed in its subconscious. Making real, loving acts from within, without expecting something in return, is a matter of course for children, so they may have understandable outbursts that can sometimes be rather painful to someone else who is not at all mindful of what is going on. The child will then be stamped "as bold as brass," but it will be quite right, most of the time.

In opening a two-way relationship with the ADHD child, this matter will play a big role. Do not play ego games, for instance by saying: "If you do that, mummy will be very sad." There is an American expression for this: a guilt trip, making the other per-son feel guilty or responsible for an unpleasant situation. Do not hold a hidden agenda, like sending the child out of the room to do something fatuous just to get some rest yourself. When you do this, the first bit of trust will go up in smoke, and the child will (once more) withdraw into its own safe little world. Remain quiet, honest, and respectful in your behavior, even if this costs you a lot of effort. Really, the child will pick it up, and it will mir-ror itself to it.

Although we need to watch this issue of trust extra carefully, immediately a question comes up: Is this really so out of the or-dinary, this need to really mutually trust each other? This does not only apply to dealing with socially handicapped kids, does it? Don't we all want to be approached in an open and honest way? Is not trust one of the highest values and virtues in human relationships? Doesn't the child hold a life-size mirror up to us, regarding this issue?

The occurrence of ADHD can be seen as a symptom of this day and age. A symptom that is symbolic of our wrong, immature attitudes, our lack of attention, our lack of honesty and lack of openness. It is the writing on the wall!

School and Home: Healthy Limits or Straitjacket?

In daily life, children need structure, a "box" with windows wide open, and many options to play. The ADHD child in particular thrives within certain limits that feel comfortable and safe. This approach works satisfactorily for all parties involved only if this kind of box is offered in a manner that shows respect for the child's own ways. This applies not only to the situation at home, but also at school. There are certain kinds of educational systems and schools that offer better coaching and more freedom for ADHD children, such as Montessori and Waldorf schools. Of course, choosing the best schooling for your child depends on many factors, and there is no way of knowing beforehand that the choice will eventually work out all right. There are regular schools with teachers and structures where ADHD children can develop well, whereas in some alternative institutions the child just does not hit it off with the teachers or the structure is too for the ADHD child, so that the situation gets completely out of hand there.

For the parents it is not always easy to see what is wise in the choice of a proper educational institution. My wife and I followed, for the most part, our own intuition and stories we heard from other parents concerning the schools we sent our children to. As a parent, one should not be afraid in any way to investigate and examine any claims of abuse, controversy, or misunderstanding, and to discuss everything openly with the children as well as with the teachers and headmaster.

In choosing the school there are many factors to consider, including:

- The type of school and the reputation of the teachers
- The location with regard to the child's own home
- The road from home to school—bicycling, by tram, train, school bus, or taken by the parents, busy or dangerous traffic on the way
- The child's personal reaction to the whole situation at school and its surroundings.

Everything needs to be considered; the pros and cons to be compared. But one of the most important things is letting the child feel that he or she is being heard and the child's opinion is respected. I have found it always striking how yielding and grown-up children will react when engaged in this process.

Healthy environmental factors will also enhance a reliable and positive framework in the direct situation at home. As early as infancy and well into puberty, we can—as much as possible, of course—work with these factors to contribute to harmony, in the most extensive meaning of the word. For instance, try consulting a color therapist who can advise you regarding the colors of the child's clothing, and the lighting, furniture, and walls of the child's room, empathetically involving the child in the eventual selection.

Of course, it does not need to be amicable all the time, but this kind of details do have their subtle impact, whether we like it or not. That is why we should make better use of it in a positive way!

Get That Body Moving!

Naturally, every ADHD child needs a daily dose of body movement, which can use up a lot of energy. This provides satisfaction and discharge. The physical exercise not only needs to be encouraged, but to be coached and kept up with as well. It should be just as self-evident as daily eating and drinking, so there must be time scheduled for exercise in the daily program. It would be nice if the school could integrate this, but if this is not possible, a parent or a coach could work with the child, preferably on an activity that appeals to the child, of course. One child will be completely fascinated by running or swimming, while the other will go for a team sport. Unfortunately, some sports clubs or extracurricular teams mainly offer activities no more than once or twice a week, while the ADHD child must have this kind of exercise on a daily basis. Of course it is a matter of age, but from the moment a child is able to make its own choice and is passionate about a certain kind of sport or game (physical, no computer games!), it is essential to encourage this wherever you can.

A good alternative exercise to do at home is the Sun Salutation exercise. Parents could do this with their child(ren) in the morning, before breakfast. The Sun Salutation is a kind of yoga workout, with a range of consecutive, flowing movements that will train the whole body, inside and outside. The practice takes just ten minutes, including relaxation afterwards, and there is no need for any equipment; it can be learned without effort. Any form of coercion should be avoided, because that would only work the wrong way around. Most basic yoga books cover this exercise but I suggest the fully illustrated description of the Sun Salutation in *Integral Yoga Hatha* by Sri Swami Satchidananda (New York: Holt, Rinehart and Winston, 1970). It is a large format book that is easy to learn from and the photos of this accomplished, elderly yogi show the perfect form and ease of the postures.

Stimulation, motivation, perseverance and endurance—those are the keys to success!

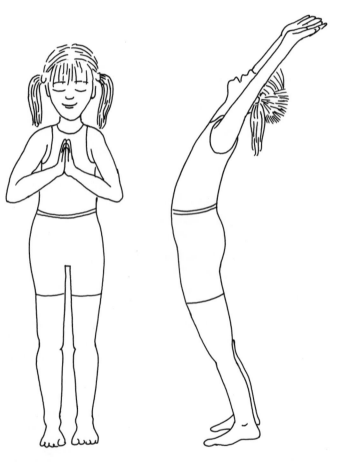

1. Breathing in and out   2. Breathing in

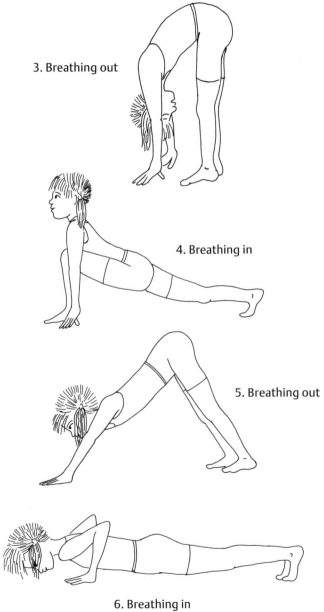

3. Breathing out

4. Breathing in

5. Breathing out

6. Breathing in

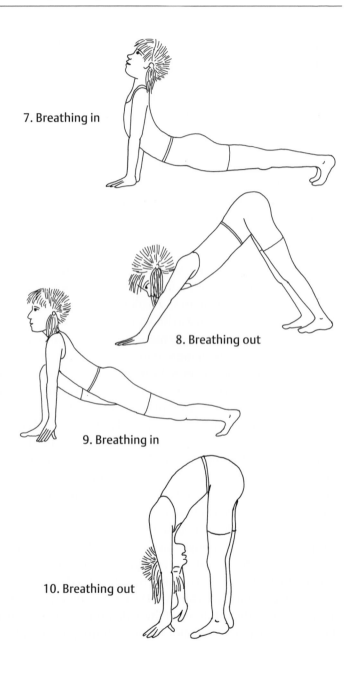

7. Breathing in

8. Breathing out

9. Breathing in

10. Breathing out

5 GETTING CLOSER
Methods

> We should always keep in mind that with ADHD—as with so many other ailments or disorders—it is more than just taking one or more pills a day that will do the job. It is clear that mutual trust— with a lot of patience and love—should be an important starting point in coaching an ADHD child at home. In this chapter, we will fix our attention upon the therapeutic methods we can choose, in order to work these into everyday life. For in practice, it turns out that many parents of children with ADHD eventually need professional support.

Various new methods have been developed, which offer structure and methods for both educators and children, in order to turn ADHD into a fascinating challenge. These will be highlighted here, with reference to books in the recommended reading list on page 107, containing more elaborated manuals on the subject, or web sites with more information. Those who are interested may delve deeper into the matter and, if desired, use the method or product. This list will certainly not be complete; these approaches and methods are still evolving.

Keep in mind when considering books about the subject and related products: everyone tries to make you think they have the answer, and every company considers its own product to be the most fantastic and effective! Fortunately, most of us are rather down-to-earth and will be able to see through this. Because it remains to be seen what is practicable, and of course there is the cost as well. Most alternative methods and products will not be compensated, even though there are good results. Unfortunately, only for this reason it is enough for regular therapists not to adopt them. In a research article by L. E. Arnold (1998), twenty-four alternative therapies for ADHD were compared to the regular approach. Although some of these therapies were promising, the study concluded that not enough thorough scientific research had been done in order to recommend them. Another disadvantageous outcome of this research was that because of the use of these methods, a good, effective, regular therapy was postponed. Essentially, such an outcome is very regrettable, because many health professionals ended up downplaying alternative therapies when some of these could have complemented an established treatment protocol.

The use of sound and music, which we will explore in this book, is not included in this list of twenty-four therapies. One of the reasons is that sound therapy is often applied as a support of, or supplementary to, other methods. Secondly, sound therapy has not been used until recently for ADHD or any specific ailment, for that matter

All the methods described here will only succeed when done with the utmost loving care and patience, which will always be the essential core.

It is also a good idea to combine the methods mentioned here with sound therapy—an interesting challenge, for all involved, parents and therapists!

---

1. The traditional approach: psychologist, medicines, neurofeedback
2. The creative approach: art therapy
3. Psychological approach, combination of methods
4. Energy work
5. Supplements
6. Sound therapy

The Traditional Approach

The regular approach for ADHD consists of psychological coaching and medication. When a child has ADHD, he or she will often show related anomalies, which makes it more difficult to find a proper treatment. Often, a prescription of medicine like Ritalin®

or Concerta®[15] will be suggested, in order to make the child more "manageable," but most people will agree that this is a provisional rather than a permanent solution. After all, the cause of the problem will not be addressed with these medicines—only the symptoms. In the last ten years the rate of intake of medicines by children has multiplied, especially children with autism and ADD/ADHD. Exact numbers are hard to find, and these vary in different countries.[16]

Health practitioners have been under fire for prescribing medicines too freely to ADHD children; many feel the doses appear to be too high as well. There is still very little known about the long-term effects of these medicines. There is also too little supervision afterwards in the use of these medicines.[17]

A prescription of medicine may offer in many cases the necessary help and/or could give parents who cannot cope with the situation some temporary relief. Still, it will become obvious that medication will not solve the causes of the problem: they do not heal.

Ritalin has been in existence for more than sixty years, and will be effective in 80 to 85 percent of patients, according to the manufacturer. The effective ingredient is methylphenidate, which is effective only short term in Ritalin, meaning that it needs to be taken several times a day. Next, there is Concerta, with the same effective ingredient, but in a slower release form. Moreover, it has an advantage over Ritalin: after the medicine has lost its efficacy, the child doesn't suffer an intensified relapse. There is another new, effective medicine, Strattera® (effective ingredient is atomoxetine HCl), that works on the line of conduct (hyperactivity and attention deficit). Unfortunately, this medicine still is ten times as expensive as the other two, and it is not yet reimbursed by Medicare. Naturally, there are many more medicines that are being used with ADHD, such as Dixarit®, Oxazepam®, and Clomipranin®, to name a few, but the use of this kind of medicine is certainly not without risk. Apparently, for instance, some children using long-term Ritalin showed physical growth slowing down to one centimeter less than average per year. Also, children who could not tolerate the medication long-term, or just stopped taking it, experienced proper weight maintenance problems, as well as anxiety and sleep disorders. With long-term medication like this, it makes you wonder if the medicine is not worse than the disease.[18]

On the other hand, there are fortunately many stories of people who can tell that their children, after using medication, were able to function much better, without noticeably weird side effects.

In many countries, Ritalin has not been registered officially for prescription to children under six. Still, some physicians will prescribe it for young children, mostly when the effectiveness of psychosocial therapy is proven inadequate. Still, the dose to start with will always be very low, sometimes only 3 to 4 milligrams a day, which apparently is enough for some to feel an improvement.[19] Concerning the psychosocial approach: we all know that the effects of this for the better part depend on the skills and experience of the attending therapist, as well as the mutual bond of confidentiality between therapist, child, and parents. Luckily, these knowledgeable, experienced therapists do exist! And a good therapist will also be open to any input from parents and teachers in relation to other ways of treatment, as described below.

Neurofeedback

When you have neurofeedback therapy, you are connected, through little sensors at your fingertips and/or skull, to a machine with a monitor that continually measures the effect that a certain kind of administered treatment or suggestion has. Through a selection procedure, the therapist may choose which signals appear to be beneficial, or make you feel pleasant and relaxed. Over the course of time, this therapy fosters a response that makes it very easy to obtain excellent results with just very light stimuli.

Neurofeedback goes a long way back, but direct methods aimed at children with neurological disorders have not been in practice that long. Usually, there are two kinds of neurofeedback used: the classical EEG-biofeedback, and the Chaos-control neurofeedback.[20] Modern afflictions such as stress, fatigue, depression, and hyperactivity can also have their repercussions on the brain. Martin Wuttke, one of the leading neurofeedback specialists, and founder of the Neurotherapy Centers in the US, developed a neurofeedback training program to help harmonize the brain frequencies. With his method, a lot of the noise in the head is reduced, so the brain will be able to recover its natural balance. Wuttke says about the starting period of this new development, "The results were phenomenal. I had permanently 35 patients available, who I could treat twice every day. The successes were—and still are—rather spectacular. With a lot of the 'endemics' of this era, like chronic fatigue, ADHD and addiction, the percentage of recovery has been around seventy to eighty percent."

It is not so easy to find a reliable neurofeedback therapist, so it seems. So it is important to shop first, for instance on the internet, before going ahead with someone. An example of the many web sites with further information can be found at www.neuro-feedback.com and www.brainquiry.com.

The Creative Approach

Within the regular psychological and psychiatric health care, creative therapy meanwhile has acquired its own place. In coaching ADHD children, some special ways of treatment are already in practice, as well. These carry great promise, in view of the excellent results.

Children's drawings can be very useful, especially while mapping any disturbances, because almost every child will be able to express itself through a scrawl or color experiment. Other than that, the child can, by being coached in this, obtain more inner structure and awareness of certain patterns and habits. Some therapists claim that even past-life impressions may come up and be processed.

BASIC DRAWING, IN SMALL STEPS FROM POLARITY TO REST

With the following exercise, you coach the child through a simple drawing, even if it's just a line being extended in small steps.[21] You need only a piece of paper and a drawing tool that the child likes.

1. Draw a line in the center of your paper.
2. What does this little line need? (Here often comes an impulsive response.)
3. All right, I see you are making a whole bunch of little lines around it! (Provide encouragement along the way.)
4. Now draw a connection between the line and the other little ones.
5. I see you are making the connection, well done!
6. Can you now make a very slow animal out of this?
7. That's nice, OK, now you can color the inside.
8. What's his name? That's a funny name!

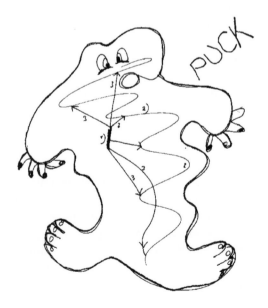

9. Could you write that next to it?
10. What is Puck (the name the child gave the animal) good at?
11. What is he bad at doing?
12. What does Puck feel now?
13. What is Puck thinking right now?
14. What would Puck really like to do now?
15. Now try to draw that around Puck, OK?

In a few clearly defined and easy to follow small steps—from a "stupid little line" developing into a kind of comic strip, this exercise works on several levels. The slow animal stands in polarity against the nervous, hyperactive ADHD child. With this imaginative, "slow down" program, the child can dive into the beneficial world of coloring and imagine itself in the personal qualities of Puck. It teaches the child how to identify with a living being and finally give it a place in a fitting environment.

THE CHAIN OF BEADS

This exercise helps with concentration and short-term memory. You need a piece of paper, crayons, colored markers, or Cray-pas (oil pastels); the latter is actually best for mixing up the colors at the end of the session. If you want to use paint instead, that's fine, too; use nontoxic tempera or poster paints. Have plenty of water available to clean the brush between colors or use three different brushes, one for each color. Always keep in mind the child's limitations and adapt the kinds of materials you use accordingly.

1. With a pencil, pen, or crayon, have the child draw a nice undulating line on the paper.
2. Have the child choose only three colors from his or her box of crayons or other type of colored marker or poster paints, and then ask the child to close the box and put it aside. The child may also choose randomly, with eyes shut. Make it fun!
3. Now have the child decide which color is number 1, which is number 2, and which is number 3.

4. Explain to the child, "With these colors you are going to make a drawing of a beautiful necklace, but you have to use the colors in order: 1-2-3."
5. Help the child stay mindful of the order of colors he or she uses while encouraging the child to come up with any beautiful shapes for the big and small beads.
6. When the chain is ready, have the child mix all three colors softly together in the area around the necklace to fill up the picture.

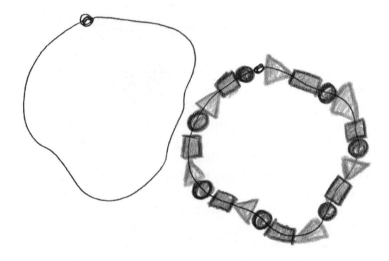

This drawing session is intended to help the child learn about creating order and making choices. In mixing the colors in the surrounding area, greater restraint is required than in the interchanging of colors in the beads and controlling the bead shapes. It may be that the ADHD child will be so over-enthusiastic that he or she looses control of the crayon or, and colors over the necklace, to then be perplexed that the necklace is gone. That's OK, because you tell the child that the necklace just lies beneath this blanket of colors. Help the child to finish the edges neatly, so it becomes a box, a blanket or a fur. Improvise so that the drawing experience is satisfying to the child.

This method is adapted from the work of Rudolf Steiner, "father" of Anthroposophy. It alternates two-dimensional drawing with colors, like the one described above, with three-dimensional expression, such as concentration exercises that involve working with massive brass bars of one centimeter in diameter, sometimes with balls at the ends. The brass rod is a symbol of communication; think of the use of copper in water pipes and electric appliances. The child is given sets of controlled movements to perform with the brass, while the teacher and the child say a verse such as "The sun is rising, the sun is setting, the sun goes up, and goes down again." With more children, we can also work on structure, like jointly shaping balanced geometrical figures in space.

For more information, visit www.genezendtekenen.nl or e-mail lisaborstlap@zonnet.nl.

Psychological Approach, Combined Methods

The following four approaches use a combination of methods which, combined, work very well and effectively.

INTEGRATED CHILD'S CORE METHOD (ICCM)
This complete approach is based on insights from Western psychology and Eastern techniques such as massage (an adaptation of Do-in, acu-massage you can use on your own body; in this case the parent or attendant will perform the massage on the child), and a change in diet and food preparation. A third, essential aspect is how one interacts with the child and the adaptation of the child's environment. These are in fact all rather simple items everybody is familiar with, and which most find easy to integrate. This makes this method so ideal. Personally, I think the most important part is that this holistic approach has led to very good results already! The booklet *Beyond ADHD* describes this method in detail. See also *Discovering Successful Pathways in Children's Development*.

THE DAVINCI METHOD
www.DaVinciMethod.com

Garret LoPorto, originator of this method, made good use of the new popularity of good old Leonardo, who, according to Lo-Porto, was the embodiment of lateral thinking, a way to look at a problem from various points of view. The DaVinci approach is very fresh and unorthodox. LoPorto's idea is that people with ADD and ADHD have an average of 20 percent higher IQ than the rest of us. He claims that such people have the DaVinci temperament, including this lateral way of thinking, that they can use to solve problems more easily. We find these people among inventors, entrepreneurs, pioneers, researchers, and artists. Accordingly, LoPorto gives clues how to develop this lateral thinking. So he approaches ADHD rather as an asset than a disorder! You can take advantage of it, provided you approach it in the right way. He claims that his method can generate geniuses. By having them solve ingenious MENSA-riddles as a kind of daily workout, the child's IQ can be raised within a very short period.

ADD TO C3 KIDS
www.addtoc3kids.com

Here, "C3" stands for "Cool, calm and collected." This method, conceived by an American mother of a son with ADD, is mainly based on change and adaptation of food, added supplements, and refraining from the usual prescribed medicines. She wrote some very popular booklets (see reading list on page 00), which can be downloaded from the internet, and which contain a number of remarkable recommendations. Her approach is actually one big indictment of the big pharmaceutical companies, which, even against the advice of the FDA, secure their gigantic sales of ADHD medicine by financing scientific research. This brings the impartiality of such research into question. The recommended supplements are distributed worldwide, through the web site, at a 25 to 50 percent discount.

WEBCAER

www.caer.com

Another medicine-free therapy is described in the book by psychologist Lawrence Weathers, *ADHD: A Path to Success.* Here, there are no diet or supplements, but the method is being taught in Spokane, WA, in an intensive three- to five-day workshop, where parents and children work together. Dr. Weathers bases his method on his own personal struggle and eventual victory over ADD. His starting point is to find how the children themselves look at the "problem," and then show how this can give the parents a better picture of how the child's mind works. A huge 92 percent of the families rated the results as outstanding to excellent. Afterwards, Dr. Weathers developed an on-line method, called WebCAER (Computer Aided Emotional Restructuring), and he wrote a book from which the first six chapters can be downloaded for free. This method works for both children and adults.

Energy Work

Because ADHD has a lot to do with the energy distribution system, therapies that deal directly with this system, like the one described here, will have a very direct effect.

FREQUENCIES OF BRILLIANCE

www.frequenciesofbrilliance.com

"Frequencies of Brilliance" is a kind of "energy healing," developed by Christine Day some 20 years ago. It is a healing process that occurs over a number of sessions. In this process, all body cells are being reprogrammed, so it can function much better. But this transformation process is not only physical; the healing and structuring will take place on all levels so that mentally there will also be more structure. Meanwhile, there have already been very good results with this rather unknown method, with ADHD children. There is a group of certified practitioners who work with this method; they can be found at the general web site.

Food Supplements

I have already explained that the lack of certain food substances can contribute to the development of ADHD, especially in young children. These deficiencies happen much more often than most people think. So, supplying these deficiencies will be a logical step in re-establishing the balance in a child.

ORTHO-MOLECULAR APPROACH
Starting from the fact that many ADHD children show a demonstrable lack of essential nutrients, various food supplements have been developed that may be effective combined with other methods. In ortho-molecular medicine the principle is to consider the human being as a whole; hence a medicine should be holistic in nature, which means that it must be effective on the entire body, not just a part. These medicines and supplements are always of a natural origin.

There is an ortho-molecular food supplement, Synaptol™ (also called the "Smart Pill"), available at www.micronutra.com. It is a synergetic blend of plant extracts and nutrients, with proven benefits and no side effects. The web site gives good documentation and many positive testimonials from parents who are using it for their children. The ingredients include: *Aloe barbadensis*, tragacanth gum, beta-glucane, arabinogalactane, shitake and maitake mushroom extracts, cordycep mycella extract, glucosamine sulfate, ghatti gum and guar gum.

The makers of the supplement report that about nine out of ten children and adults with ADD/ADHD will show improvement in school performance within the first seven days. The product is shipped worldwide through the web site, with a discount for a year's supply.

Another effective product, Focus ADHD Formula® from Native Remedies (www.nativeremedies.com), is also a mixture of extracts from rather popular herbs such as *Ginkgo biloba* and *Avena sativa* (wild oats). This product is also from the United States, but is being distributed worldwide. It is often used together with a homeopathic ADD/ADHD remedy called BrightSpark®. From the web site you can also download a free e-booklet, *How to Manage Your ADHD Child*, together with your order.

Finally, in Chapter 3, note 17, I already mentioned the food supplement ConcenTrace®, which also has been tested thoroughly. This is available online at www.traceminerals.com

MAGNESIUM

Only in the last few years, science has been enriched with a huge amount of knowledge about the effects and importance of magnesium in numerous life processes in our bodies. Magnesium is the fourth most present mineral in the body, with half of it in our bones; most of the other half is in cells of tissues and organs, and only one percent is in our bloodstream. The body will do everything to keep this percentage constant. Magnesium determines the right electrolytes balance, resulting in a good metabolism (converting food nutrients into energy and building blocks for the cells, and then the discharge of waste materials) in the cells. In this process it also has a determining role in stabilizing the cell membrane.

In most people in the Western world there appears to be a sometimes alarming magnesium deficiency in the body (see Chapter 3 page 28). In 1909 the average intake of magnesium through food in the US was still 408 milligrams a day, but in 1985 this amount had gone down to just 228 mg in women and 323 mg in men. This may cause a range of various, often serious ailments and illnesses, among others that we call "civilization sicknesses." A lack of magnesium will have consequences for almost all body functions and may be—among other causes—responsible for coronary diseases, headaches and migraines, diabetes, nervous diseases, memory and brain failure, and many kinds of cancer.

The characteristic features of someone with ADHD are almost a perfect match with people who show a magnesium deficiency! So it is no surprise that with a magnesium supplement, miraculous changes for the better can happen. These findings are mainly the results of the excellent work of young professor Mark Sirrus, who after numerous researches and equations wrote his book *Transdermal Magnesium Therapy* (2006). He writes about his own and others' experiences with employing magnesium while treating mainly autistic children, but also children with other neurological disorders.

As causes of the magnesium deficiency, Dr. Sirrus cites:

- The dramatic diminishment of magnesium in our raw food.
- Over-processed food and drink that has no nutritional value.
- Most children have lost their ability to assimilate these nutrients sufficiently.
- The supplements prescribed by doctors do not have the right composition, so most of the magnesium and other elements are not absorbed at all. Especially a mineral like magnesium is very difficult to be absorbed through an oral supplement.

Loss and lack of magnesium is exacerbated by the use of alcohol, excessive amounts of caffeine, sugar, diuretics (medicines, but also diuretic herbs!), and oral contraceptives. Vaccinations may also be a cause. Other substances that stimulate loss of magnesium are: cocaine, beta-adrenergetic antagonists (used in treating excessive and uncontrolled muscle contraction), theophylin and steroids (bronchodilators used to treat asthma), thiazide, phosphates (in cola drinks), nicotine, and insulin.

There is growing evidence that a low magnesium level contributes also to storing heavy metals in the brain; a process preceding Parkinson's, multiple sclerosis and Alzheimer's diseases. There are so many clear and evident relations, that it is obvious that magnesium plays a crucial part in these as well as ADHD.

Dr. Bernhard Rimland from the Autism Research Institute (www.autismwebsite.com/ARI) researched the effects of vitamin B, combined with magnesium. He discovered, while doing interchanging double-blind and placebo-controlled tests with sixteen autistic children, that statistically there could be substantial positive results. It appears that children and adults will also sleep better when taking magnesium with supper.

Because magnesium appears to be difficult to be assimilate when taken orally,[22] the best way to administer it is by injection—which of course is not very practical with kids! There is, however, a special, pure magnesium oil, to be used while massaging the child. So it may become a part of the ICC method outlined on page 59. Another option is taking a hot bath with a little magnesium oil in the water, for at least half an hour, once every three days to begin with, and later once a week will do. There are also special magnesium bath flakes, and there is a magnesium probiotic for internal use. All the magnesium products I mentioned are available at www.globallight.net.

MINERALS FROM THE OCEAN, WITH FRESH PLANT JUICES
In the 1920s, the young Swiss pharmacist Walter Schoenberger did a lot of pioneering work with the correct preparation of beneficial plants and herbs by. The usual method of processing medicinal plants until Schoenberger's methods evolved, was to make infusions—the oldest method in the world—or prepare an alcohol-based tincture. Unfortunately, with these methods a lot of the effects are lost. Schoenberger did countless experiments, proving that only freshly made plant and herb juices have a real therapeutic value, which is just unrivaled in the effects of dried plants. He prepared his first plant juices in his mother's kitchen. After careful washing, the freshly gathered plants were hand-pressed and the juice was stored in sterilized bottles. After endless tests, in 1924 he could finally prove scientifically that it is actually these fresh plant juices that contain all nutrients in well-balanced proportions, supporting good health. Only the fresh plant contains the concentrated healing power that nature created, present in unaltered form, explained Schoenberger.

In 1927 he invented a method to naturally stabilize the fresh juices in such a manner that these could be kept for several months, even years, and thus be utilized all year long in hospitals and sanatoriums. So in 1927 he started his own little company in the Black Forest near Stuttgart, Germany. He succeeded in getting farmers to grow sufficient plants for him, like nettle, dandelion, and yarrow. This was an essential revolution in those days, when large-scale agriculture, mono-culture, and chemical pesticides were just evolving. Even today, these juices from fresh, organically grown plants and herbs are still being made and applied all over the world.

Only a decade ago, this had a special sequel. An Australian by the name of Gerry Amena developed an exceptional method that used no heat or chemicals, making not only the effects of freshly pressed plants stronger, but also enhancing their keeping qualities without loosing any effectiveness. Amena discovered how to stabilize these ingredients in his successful attempt to save his son who had terminal cancer.

During a number of months, the selected, hand-picked organic herbs are mixed with the best sea minerals, resulting in—to my knowledge—the very best food supplements ever. In terms of composition, one liter of Ocean Minerals solution equals that of a hundred liters of ocean water. The human body will absorb an incredible 98 percent of these minerals, because these are water soluble electrolytes. Science will never be able to mimic these minerals; they are a gift of nature.

The herbs that Amena uses are organically grown, and they are cut, ground, and mixed with the minerals within ten minutes after harvesting, so they are exclusively used fresh. The salt crystals provide a tiny layer around the herbs, so the freshness and effectiveness can be preserved for a very long time. This way, the herbs contain more healing power than any other brand on the market. This is the secret behind their effectiveness on a whole range of disorders. The healing properties are stabilized and preserved, because immediately after the harvest they are mixed with the minerals; they are not heated and no alcohol is used.

Independent research has shown that the herbs that are processed in Ocean Minerals have an antiinflammatory effect; they will help the body resist viruses, bacteria, and parasites in a powerful, safe and nonpoisonous way, and they have many more wholesome properties.

Together with the indispensable minerals—for instance,

there is a very well absorbable magnesium compound—and trace elements from the ocean water (which so much resembles our blood plasma), this is a product that certainly may have good results with ADHD and related behavior as well. There already have been reports from children using these minerals, on a daily basis, with good results. According to Amena, it would be an excellent idea to introduce the minerals into the school system, and to work with them in cases of autism, ADD, or ADHD. Children with ADD or ADHD can also use the plain minerals (without added herbs), if there are no other additional complaints. Amena is quite positive in his opinion that the basis of ADHD is created during pregnancy, or in the first few months after birth, because of a lack of essential minerals. In my opinion, it is a bit more complicated than that, but at least it is partly true!

In this time and age, with so many deficiencies in our food, it will always be advisable to treat ourselves and our children with the best available supplements. You can order these minerals through this www.globallight.net. Australians can order directly from Gerry Amena at: www.seamineral.com/prod.asp.

• • •

SOUND THERAPY

Many decades ago in France, Dr. Alfred Tomatis developed a listening therapy, using high frequency pulses in classical music that has been filtered in a very specific way. Listening to this kind of music results in a better functioning of the inner ear, the organ of equilibrium and hearing, as well as an increase in vital energy. Autistic children respond very well to listening to their mother's voice altered and filtered in this same way. There are listening centers in Europe and the United States that practice this therapy (www.thelisteningcenter.net), but there is also a method available for use at home. For this home therapy you need at least two CDs with filtered sound therapy music or nature sounds, and you are supposed to listen daily for about half an hour or more. While listening you can do other things like reading. The first sound therapy ("for the Walkman®") from Patricia Joudry has been enhanced and is now continued by her daughter Rafaela, based in Australia, and is available worldwide through the internet (www.soundtherapyinternational.com). Another excellent sound therapy, using the same techniques, comes from Ingo Steinbach in Germany: *The Samonas* series (www.samonas.com), distributed in the U.S. by Tools for Exploration (www.toolsforexploration.com).

London's Light and Sound Therapy Centre was founded in 1992 by Mrs. Landau, who has also worked for many years with people with learning disabilities. Initially, two practitioners in auditory integration training from the U.S. were invited to treat nine children. The improvements seen were considered sufficient to warrant making the treatment available to larger numbers of people and The Light and Sound Therapy Centre was consequently set up. Since then over 800 children and adults have been treated with the unique AIT PLUS combination treatment, which is not available anywhere else in the world. The treatment is a combination of auditory integration training (AIT), light therapy, and a sound modulation system that has a good chance of helping a child with ADHD (www.light-and-sound.co.uk).

The Mother's Voice Technique

Sound Therapy International also offers a miniature device that can be purchased for use in the home. The "Sound Therapy Converter" can be connected to a CD player or stereo and will convert any music or voice recordings into sound therapy. Now the child can listen to its own mother's voice as sound therapy through the converter. This technique offers profound healing and is an important part of the Tomatis program, especially for children with serious problems. Also available is a voice attachment that allows the child to hear its own voice through the converter as it is speaking. The converter is usually introduced after an initial period of using the CDs.

Sound Wave Energy

Another very peculiar but effective sound therapy is the sound wave energy (SWE). French-Canadian Nicole La Voie, the creator of the sound wave energy technology (vibrational frequencies), founded this therapy in 1992. She is an international lecturer and author of the book *Return to Harmony: Creating Harmony and Balance through the Frequencies of Sound.*

As a hospital X-ray technician, Nicole was exposed to harmful x-rays during her pregnancy, and her son Robert was born with many deficiencies. At the early age of five his glandular system ceased functioning. He then needed hormone replacement therapy, which improved his condition only marginally. Also, during this time, Nicole herself developed osteoporosis. Driven by these experiences, and the desire to help her son, she studied sacred geometry, Rife technology, worked with crystals, and homeopathy, became a Reiki Master, and eventually found her way to research in sound therapy. This led her to develop the system of frequencies known as Sound Wave Energy (SWE), which has healed her, her son, and many others with challenges, at all levels. Nicole is now totally committed to sharing this simple, effective technique for empowering people to support their own return to harmony. SWE frequencies are based on sacred geometry and the frequencies of minerals, vitamins, noble gases, amino acids, and hormones. These frequencies balance and harmonize the physical, emotional, mental, and spiritual bodies. The low frequencies, in the range of 15 to 33 Hertz, will sound like a cat's purr or an engine's hum; they are not musical. These different tones can help ADHD children achieve balance, so they can function much better. Find out more about Nicole La Voie's work at www.harmonyera.com.

6 REVERBERATION
How Sounds Can Help

In this chapter we will further explore sound therapy. A kind of complementary therapy for ADHD children that is still in its infancy, therapy with special sounds has not been extensively researched or documented. This does not mean, however, that we cannot go ahead with it very seriously!

Sound Massage

The word "sound" has a double meaning. We can use sounds to heal ourselves—to become sound in mind and sound in body, to become whole. And this goes much further than feeling comfortable while listening to a nostalgic tune on the radio (although there is nothing wrong with that!).

Sounds can also be very destructive. Think of loud explosions of fireworks or warfare, or literally deafening house music; also the noise of heavy traffic—cars, trains, planes, motorcycles—sometimes these constitute a continuous source of sound-environmental pollution. Almost every one of us gets a daily share of disturbing sounds, which have a tiring and chaotic effect on us. As a counterbalance for all this confusion from disturbing noise, we can choose to surround ourselves, at set times, with harmonizing, healing sounds. This may be primarily silence, or the rustling of the wind during a long walk in nature. But we can also make more specific choices, like a certain kind of sound, pitch, hummed vowels, and the like, in order to generate a very special effect.

It is possible to eventually select one or more sounds that you specifically need in order to let your energy flow freely and to make you feel healthier and happier. The same applies to people with ADHD problems.

Let us first have a look at the ways sound reaches and affects us. Sound does not only enter the body through the ears. The whole body is being resonated and vibrated by sound. The word resonance comes from the Latin *resonare,* meaning "reverberating," "re-sounding." Compare it with throwing a rock in the water, which causes great turbulence on and below the surface, expanding into all directions. This turbulence, this impulse, is harmonious in nature; witness the concentric circles around the point of impact. Likewise, a certain tone of sound can cause a similar harmonious resonance in the human energy system.

Sounds will not only work at the level of energy, but also physically. Japanese researcher Dr. Emoto demonstrated with resonance pictures what sound can do at the cellular level.[23] Our bodies consist for the most part of water, which is easily vibrated. Dr. Emoto made pictures of water crystals that had been exposed to different kinds of sound, with very obvious differing results in structure. With harmonious sounds, we see a balanced color mandala, while with chaotic sounds there is a corresponding blur.[24] So we can establish that the more harmonious the sound structure of a tone or a piece of music is, the more harmonious the outcome will be of the resonating image within our bodies. We may even go a little further and infer that the intention of the maker of the sound—for instance the one who plays the singing bowls, or even the combined intention of a whole orchestra—can make a difference in effect upon the receiver, the listener. You will probably know this from being at a performance or concert: a composition of a well-known composer can come across with a mighty beautiful energy from the orchestra, while the same piece by another orchestra can be completely ruined. This has often nothing to do with technical abilities, but more with the combined positive intention of both the conductor and the orchestra. Although this may be explained as a matter of feeling, we cannot deny the evidence. Thus, John Diamond describes in his book *Life Energy in Music* that some chemical processes at a nuclear level can only happen correctly when the person who initiates the process also has a positive mind set, while someone with a negative intention initiating the same process will not get started!

By the way, you can be assured that while recording the CD in this book, our positive intention was present for a full 100 percent!

The sounds around us obviously influence us because body fluids will resonate with these sound vibrations. The very loud and heavy sounds will not only cause the body fluids and soft tissues to resonate, but even our bone structure, including the skull. As an example I mention the well-known drone of the bass beat during house parties, which literally pierces you to the very marrow of your bones. If this goes on long enough—sometimes a couple of hours will be too much—this could permanently damage the ear, but might even damage the bone marrow and several organs such as the heart, kidneys, and liver.

Further on in this chapter—in the "Neurosonic Sounds" section—we will go further into the function of the brain, the various brain waves, and the influence of specific sound vibrations upon the brain waves and consciousness. So in that way there is also an influence. Most people do not even stop at the thought of this.

ADHD children are much more sensitive to all ways that sound can come to us from our environment, in all its variety and volumes. It is like the self-acting filter that we generally can switch on in cases of overload, does not work as adequately in them as it should. The same happens in most highly-sensitive persons. For someone who is not familiar with this it is just inconceivable how severely loud sounds will literally flood their body and mind. Actually, ADHD children can be activated or irritated by very small sounds. Unfortunately, the influence and effects of sound cannot always be estimated correctly, because some children will hide behind a wall of seeming indifference. It is as though the sounds do not affect them, and they will only react when exposed to very loud, sudden sounds; then it will almost always be a reaction of fright!

While using sounds as a therapy, such an excessive stimulus

may sometimes be necessary for a short moment, in order to shake up the child;[25] afterwards we can resume applying the more subtle tones and sounds.

Hopefully I have made it very clear that it is of the utmost importance that especially with ADHD children we need to make very conscious choices as to which sounds and music they are exposed to on a daily basis. Yes, I know, regretfully, you do not always have this choice. But still we can keep trying to utilize these options very consciously!

Sound Environment

A good way to create an agreeable, unpretentious sound atmosphere (did you catch the two meanings?) is the use of classical music as a regular background. The effectiveness is well known, although seldom used consciously.

Young children are usually very accessible to many different kinds of music. In this sense it would be a good idea to let them get acquainted with classical music at a fairly young age. Also, when choosing an instrument, it will be good to carefully consider which one suits the child. Mind you, that it is something else than the instrument that the parents think suits their child! Certain special schools, like the Waldorf schools, are handling this very well.

Also in the domain of sound environment the rule is: lead by example. When parents themselves are daily playing loud and chaotic music in the living room, don't be surprised when the children growing up in this din show disturbances of conduct at an early stage already. By the way, it is really not only classical music that is good, of course. There are other kinds of music that—provided they are played back at a modest volume—can create a very cozy atmosphere. The idea that only music from acoustic instruments would be good has long been outdated. Children at the age of eight years and older will often already have built up an aversion to classical music, because it is in their own conceit "old fashioned music" that is only played by their "stupid" parents, and from which they just need to dissociate. No, they need their own "cool"—and raving loud—music; but who is actually telling them this?

In the 1970s, new age music pioneer Steven Halpern and others produced a new kind of music that I then introduced in Europe as a kind of sound and melody for relaxation, which was completely unheard of in those days. These sounds have as characteristic features a simple melodic theme, caressing the ears and gratifying the senses, often with soft nature sounds in the background. This music was soon adopted by several institutions for the mentally and physically handicapped, and they even installed special rooms where everything was soft and smooth: the light, the colors, the floor. In my country, we named these sounds "snoozel music," and these rooms were the snoozel rooms, which are nowadays commonly used in most institutions, although—in my opinion—there still is not enough knowledge there to make an optimum use of these facilities.

Today, this music category is still called "new age." Most ADHD children like this kind of music, although some will find it too soft, or soporific. Well, that is just one of the effects of that kind of music! It can be very effective with hyperactivity, but it needs to be administered at the right place and at the right moment, of course. And by far not everything in this category is good and effective—there is a lot of chaff among the wheat. Here the muscle test that I described on page 30 can be used to find out which music will be effective for the child. Unfortunately, there is no hallmark, so you need to select this music yourself.

In the resources section of this book I list some examples in classical, new age and neurosonic music and sound that can be used effectively. You could build a collection of these, if need be, but I advise that you first borrow these from others, or select them at the library. Then, after experimenting make your own selection of sound environment where the child can feel comfortable and trusted: in the living room, in the child's own room, and even on the Walkman or iPod.

Neurosonic

After using special music to create a special sound environment in the home, we can still go one step further by using specifically designed sounds and music that can affect our brain waves—and so our consciousness. The name for this kind of music is "neurosonic." CDs with neurosonic sounds are not yet available in general record stores, but can be found in new age shops. How do these sounds actually work?

By using extra-sensitive equipment, one can measure[26] which kind of brain waves—very faint electromagnetic currents—are being produced by the brain. This is always a mixture of several stages of consciousness: beta (more than 14 Hertz, or vibrations per second), alpha (9-13 Hz), theta (4-8 Hz) and/or delta (0.5-3 Hz). In general you can say that the higher the vibratory rate, the more active the brain and our consciousness.

An example of neurosonic effects can be found at a heavy construction site. The piles are rammed into the ground with a rhythm of about one count per second, which corresponds with the brain waves in deep delta. No wonder that those old men, who are always present at such sites to watch the piling, often seem to be in a kind of trance; that is because of this rhythm! Someone in a trance will show brain waves that are mainly in delta. Also the deafening stamping at rock concerts and in discos often has this rhythm. Add to that a sound volume not a single body can resist, and the crowd gets completely out of its minds, The results of this are sometimes frightening, now, or at a later age. And this can go a lot further than a serious hearing loss: brain failure, disturbance of balance, serious lack of concentration. It is comparable with the long-term results of drug abuse, something that today is once more very topical. For it appears that so-called harmless drugs like marijuana when used for a long time can cause serious brain damage after all (just like excessive use of alcohol, by the way!).[27]

A typical brain scan of an ADHD child will show a peak in beta waves, with little highlights in alpha and theta. Delta is almost always completely absent, even during sleep, while usually in most people during sleep, or in a trance, mainly delta waves will be present, often with an occasional peak in alpha or theta. The aim of applying neurosonic sounds will then be to introduce certain brain wave patterns into the brain through a sophisticated mixture of sound vibrations beneath the music, in order to cause the brain waves to resonate with these special patterns and accordingly create a new mindset.

To accomplish this, specific techniques were created. When, for instance, you bring a constant tone of 100 Hertz into your left ear, and one of 104 Hertz into the right ear, a "phantom wave" will resonate in your brain of 104 minus 100 is 4 Hertz, that is a theta vibration. This technique has also been used on the CD with this book (tracks 1, 3, 9, and 10).

An ADHD child which mainly lives "in beta," and then listens to a track like that with a neurosonic brain wave synchronization, will not instantly go into a deep, relaxed state of mind. It might even conjure up some resistance at first. It needs time to get used to the sensation. So be a little patient and administer the sounds in small doses and without any coercion. In due time, the child will, when it realizes that this feels nice indeed, even ask for it.

Usually, a neurosonic sound will have a combination of several wave patterns, in order to invoke a specific reaction and corresponding state of mind in the brain. As an example, the ADHD child could listen before bedtime to the following sequence: at the start of the recording it would be 30 percent beta – 30 percent alpha – 20 percent theta – 20 percent delta, and then gradually, in the course of half an hour, shift to a proportion of 0 percent beta – 40 percent alpha – 20 percent theta – 40 percent delta.[28] This would make the child have a much better, deeper, and healthier sleep. Like I said, this will not happen overnight, and not every child will react the same way, either. But soundtracks like that could also be applied during the day, as a break, to get a short but restful time-out. A therapist could use these sounds as background during a session when he communicates with the child (like tracks 6 and 10).

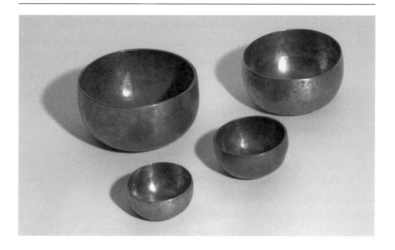

Singing Bowls

As a sound environment for the CD, we selected yet something else; namely, sounds that are practically unknown: singing bowls. Singing bowls have a very special place in sound therapy, because they produce extremely pure ranges of overtones. It is a pity that most people do not know this yet. But in this case it is perhaps an advantage, because the child will not immediately categorize a sound that it does not recognize at once as stupid or soft, and so on. In other words: the sounds will be neutral in the child's ears; the child has not saved them yet in his or her memory/experience databank, so the experience will be pure and effective. And then, when there are positive results and good feelings after listening, there will soon be an inclination to listen more often! In some of the singing bowl tracks on the CD we built in neurosonic effects, enhancing the effectiveness.

Singing bowls, sometimes combined with other instruments and/or nature sounds, have a wonderful effect—full of wonders![29] Their sound is round and warm. It is like a very comfortable blanket draped around you. And this is just what the ADHD child, thinking it lacks a safe, trusted environment, needs. The sounds will be perceived as a structure, making it feel good. And, as explained further on, a lot of this music can be used very well together with one or more other therapies. So far, this has not been used very often, and every parent or therapist will need to find his own direct application by experimenting. It would be good to keep a journal of these experiments, and also to share experiences with others, maybe in a parent's group or association for ADHD children. You are also encouraged to contact me directly and tell me about your experiences.

In the next chapter we are going to put the theory into practice!

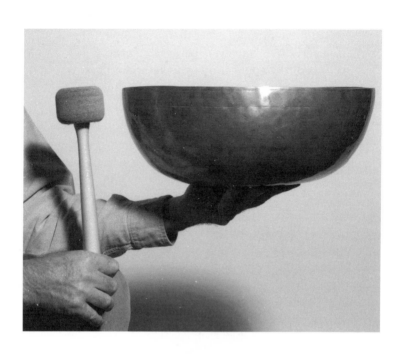

7 PRACTICE
A Promise

We have recognized the signposts of ADHD. We have learned to listen and to exchange. We gained more insight and understanding in the ways ADHD can develop and which processes may play a part. We now have also new hopes that, apart from suppressing medicines, there are several alternative methods and solutions that, often when combined, may really show good results. Finally, we were introduced into the magic world of sound massage: unique and versatile, but still not used very often. In this last chapter, we will how can we employ sounds throughout the development and education of ADHD children, coercion in a fun and light way The accessory CD contained with this book will play the most important role in this.

Healing sounds . . . it all sounds very promising, literally figuratively. Not only can sounds and music play a supporting role, when combined with other methods, in helping the ADHD child, but also we can experiment with the use of the sounds as a primary treat. Further on we will describe the various tracks on the CD, and the different ways in which they may be used, for instance, one track programmed on repeat, or a combination of two or more tracks in a specific playback sequence. There is a multitude of possibilities, of which just a few are further elaborated on in this book. Experiments by parents, teachers, and therapists—and the child's feedback—will eventually supply more information.

When you look at the track list for the CD, it will be clear that this is certainly not just soft new age music, on the contrary. Often we work with contrast and counterpart, for instance first a rather loud, profound sound of a gong, followed by much smoother, harmonizing overtone sounds, or a square, rhythmic sound like a heartbeat, with a mixed-in pattern of sounds in a free and varying intensity. Playing with these sounds, moods, and rhythms gives us many therapeutic possibilities, even if we have little experience with them. A therapist can of course work much more directly and intensely with these sounds, and may on the grounds of his collective experience develop—in the course of time—a complete, special sound program. Here also it would be desirable that eventually these experiences could be exchanged between therapists!

A promising wish. A wishful promise.

Listening to the CD

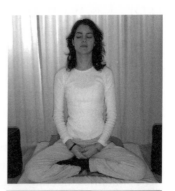

In order to make the best use of the CD recordings, it is important to know that these will only be effective when listening through good sound equipment, the loudspeakers being the most important factor. In any case you want to use good, big speakers, to be positioned in two ways: either on both sides of the child (sitting or lying down, or at the child's feet when lying down (see pictures). A surround system is of course also an excellent option.

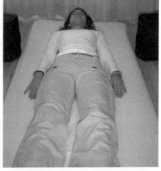

It does not make sense to listen to the CD with headphones. Because we work with particular instruments, like gongs and singing bowls, the use of small, weak speakers creates little to no effect. The speakers need to be able to reproduce a minimum of 50 watts of music capacity. Only

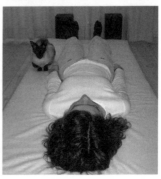

then will the surrounding air be vibrated enough so it can be literally felt in the body, and that really is the aim here. So a good quality sound system (not a portable little player) is essential for the eventual effects. Such a system is also needed because the kind of sounds on the CD are easily distorted when using inferior speakers, so this can result in distorted reproduction.

Toning

"Toning" is the singing of vowels and sounds, which can also effect healing by providing a soothing discharge for the emotions. You will first need to practice the technique before bringing it into practice. Children often like this kind of singing very much. Consciously using sound can work little miracles with emotional blockages. In the list below, you will see with each vowel a number of qualities that have been experimentally determined. Still, it's good to keep in mind that these are general patterns that might not work exactly the same with everybody. They are general tendencies that we can use when dealing with emotions.

When working with these sounds, you may find that the pitch is of less importance here, although you may couple, for instance, the AH vowel to the pitch of the heart area, the tone of F, which has been recorded on the CD in track 7.

UH (as in true) grounding, more solid in your body, calming, relaxing, feeling of security
OH (as in coach) awareness, better self-image and identity, individuality, stomach area
AH (as in maharishi) reaching out to the world, feelings from the heart, feel like creating space
EY (as in may) being able to express yourself, also listening to the other, communication
EE (as in see) energy, waking up from lethargy, mental and physical endurance

MM more balance and harmony, more room in the head, very relaxing

HRAIIIM (hrahiiimmm) expression and neutralizing of sorrow and suffering

EEM-NN-EH head, throat, neck, and shoulders relax, being able to express yourself

AH-MMAH opens the heart, provides room for expression of feelings

OH-MMAEEEH centering, connecting head and feet, and facilitates expression

HUUMUUMM creates a deep grounding and solidity, together with inner tranquility; can also be used when the child is fearful

You can sing the sound UAIMMM to direct the energy flow in an upward direction, while the sound MIAUUUUU will bring the energy from your head into the body. The latter is important for people who are living too much in their heads (worriers as well as dreamers).

CD CONTENTS

The CD contains the sounds of Tibetan singing bowls, gongs, and other special instruments—as well as vocal chords—which have been demonstrated to have a special effect, physically as well as mentally. Sounds make up a universal language that every human can understand and feel. As such, the CD has mainly an accompanying function during processes like therapy, communication, activation, or relaxation. But the CD may also be used primarily to generate certain effects, and to submerge the child in a warm and pleasant sound bath. It is already known that these natural sounds can have special effects, but in addition we used neurosonic effects (in tracks 1, 3, 9 and 10), subtle manipulations in the sounds, influencing the brain waves of the listener, for instance, slowing down their vibration into a deep, relaxed state. With ADHD children this can work very effectively. And when they realize themselves that it works, they will be motivated to listen more often to these sounds.

Although of course you can also just listen to the CD as a pleasant background, it really is designed as a tool for certain purposes with a clear intent, outlined in this chapter.

The different tracks can, sometimes in certain combinations, be used for various goals. They are long enough for use during therapy sessions and such, if needed by programming tracks on repeat. Or they can be played back repeatedly, or in certain combinations (see further on for some examples). You can ask the child: "Do you want to hear it one more time?"

The child will preferably lie down comfortably, or sit with the support of soft cushions. His or her own cozy listening spot would be ideal, a kind of private snoozel space. In any case, everything should be soft; there must also be ample room for moving around freely and playful dancing with some of the tracks. While listening, try to minimize the chance for interference or disturbances such as friends who drop by, the telephone or door bell, or anything like that.

The sound volume is very important. It should not be too loud, otherwise it could probably be too threatening; but it should also not be too low, because then there will not be enough reverberation in the body (see Chapter 7, Listening to the CD, page 82). In some situations, like during a therapy session, it might be necessary to turn up the volume for a little while in order to get a process going.

All recordings are aimed at positively influencing the concentration and other problems that ADHD children experience. The CD is certainly not meant as a substitute for medication prescribed by a physician, but as an attempt to obtain positive changes by means of harmonic sounds, and hopefully, over the course of time, to reduce the use of medicines.

TRACKS DESCRIPTION

1. Tibetan singing bowls: acoustical neurosonic signal (gong) and rhythmic movement

Soundscape: Melodic rhythms and pulses, with an accompanying singing bowl in continuous keynote, with deep ± 2 Hz (deep delta) brain wave synchronization, with also a left/right signal.
Objective: Relaxation by influencing the brain wave rhythms through sound interference.
Explanation: The brain sends impulses to all muscles in the body, for a complete relaxation that is really perceptible. The melodic and rhythmic impulses pass on sound structures to various parts of the body, causing a deeply relaxing resonance within.

Left and right brain halves are synchronized by the sound interference of the left and right channel, and the brain wave rhythm shifts toward alpha and theta, with a delta wave deep down. With good loudspeakers you can literally feel the relaxing drone in you body, a extraordinary experience. Perhaps the first few times you should play back this track a little softer, and when you are accustomed to the sound you can turn up the volume. So this track can be used to reduce unrest and tension. When working with this track, help lead the child's attention to the various sounds: "Do you hear the difference between left and right? What do you feel now in your body?"

2. Chinese wind chime and Burmese gong: timeless movements

Soundscape: Waves in a free rhythm, combined with intensities (stimuli) from the gong, in a steady, rhythmic pulsation.

Objective: Alternately letting go of the physical, to then incarnate once more into the body.

Explanation: The layers of the low Burmese gong have a grounding effect and gives a feeling of being in contact with the body and the earth —because of its deep and repeated rhythmic sound. It is also soothing to the brain because the gong alternates left and right while the rustling of the wind will dislodge the mind from the physical, The spirit is released in a free and timeless movement, to then always return again into the physical body. The clusters of the wind chime cause an interchanging tensing and relaxing of the physical system.

Coach the child in perceiving and following attentively these sound movements. With a good sound system (certainly when using surround sound) you can even discern back and front dimensions. The subtle sounds of the wind gongs are clearly discernable somewhere high in the room, and will comfortably arrange themselves around you, when you are lying down or sitting in between the speakers.

It may happen that children at first feel an aversion to listening to this track. They will miss the anchor points to hold on to, making them feel like they are floating in space. The children need to be coached very carefully, so after some time they will be able to let go and let it just happen. And then they will feel fine afterwards!

Observe well how the child's body reacts and coach where

needed. In no instance should the heavy sounds get across as threatening or somber, so if needed give subtle hints like: "Impressive, do you feel these vibrations inside your body? Special, huh?"

3. Cymbals and Chinese gong: experiencing extreme frequencies

Soundscape: Melodic movements, high frequencies (energy!) with the gong in regular subsound pulsations. In the second half of this track you will only hear the light sounds of the cymbals, making you drift into a restful dreamland.

Objective: The child is allowed for once to be completely him- or herself, in a dream world of sounds, with high frequency energy activation and recharging of the brain.

Explanation: The symbolism of earth (gong) and starry sky (cymbals) results in solid ground, with openness to the outside world.

The extreme difference in frequencies will connect the body to the spiritual world.

4. Wooden xylophone and Burmese gong: experiencing rest and movement

Soundscape: Wood, percussion, rhythmic movements of ocean waves, with the gong as a central quietude.

Objective: Soothing and centering; bodily experiencing the sounds.

Explanation: During the wood sounds one can move along rhythmically, perhaps clapping hands or dancing along, or make boxing movements as a kind of aggression release. During the gong sounds you may move your arms in a graceful way. This track is meant for the physical experience of contrasts and for learning to control your own energy.

There will also be resting points where the movements may be stopped completely, as a contrast, to then again gloriously move on in your own ways of expression. Some children like this moving along with sounds, but others find it odd to do and let go. Try to transmit that it can bring a liberating feeling and that this can make you feel much more free and good, something that ADHD children so often are missing.

5. Marimba and wind chime: mobile and restful

Soundscape: Melodic and rhythmic movement; the wind chime has a liberating and flowing effect.
Objective: Alternately tensing and relaxing, experiencing the difference, free movement.
Explanation: The marimba gives jazzy impulses to move about in the room, while the gongs provide the contrast of letting go, to eventually relax again and return to the state of rest.

This track is also good to use with visualizations, either guided or spontaneous. You can also let the child tell his or her own story with the sounds. This may provoke a lot of emotions, but also clarity, for the child as well as for the coach.

The track is also suitable for free movement, slow and flowing, like a kind *of tai chi* exercise. There is no melody to hold on to; the sounds are whirling through the room, emphasizing playfulness and freedom. Eventually, you may continue directly to track 6.

6. Kalimba, Chinese gong and Tibetan singing bowl: relaxing in pentatonics

Soundscape: Melodic kalimba, from a firm touch toward peace and rest. Now and then a singing bowl comes in. The sounds are moving around in the room, and the sound volume does also vary.
Objective: The pentatonic range (i.e., a melodic scale of 10 notes without half tones) creates a lively and liberating feeling in the body.
Explanation: Danny Becher describes his experience with this track: "All heavily handicapped people who I have worked with, and all who came in touch with the instrument (kalimba), expe-

rienced the cheerfulness and openness of these sounds, relaxed pretty fast, and felt at home. Concerning the muscle tone they had in their bodies, the pentatonic scale works as a contrast with the polarizing effects. This is clearly a track with specific opportunities for therapists, but laypersons can listen as well, to get a delicious stimulant followed by relaxation." This track goes from unstructured towards an actually recognizable melody line.

7. Voice and overtones: searching for and discovering the hidden sounds behind the voice

Soundscape: Voice and overtones.

Objective: To create a physically and mentally relaxing sound space, and relocate consciousness to another, timeless dimension.

Explanation: This track is a special exercise in listening. The child can go searching for the hidden sounds behind the voice. The physical resonance of the voice singing harmonic overtones in a whistle-like melody creates more room inside the body of the listener. Here we are using a basic tone F, which is connected with the heart chakra that is so often completely blocked in ADHD children. You can sing along, together with the child, with an MMM, or UH or AH. You will often get surprising feedback on what the child senses and perceives while doing this! A long track, almost ten minutes, it makes the listener lose all sense of time. Some children perceive it as just a few minutes, while others think it is half an hour. Explain beforehand clearly to the child what overtones are.

8. Crystal singing bowls and Burmese gong

Soundscape: Crystal singing bowls and Burmese gong.

Objective: Healing through polarities. Experiencing the continuous changing of inhalation and exhalation, expansion and contraction.

Explanation: Crystal bowls produce sounds like harmonious

constellations with specific effects on the emotional body. This track creates a sense of timeless relaxation, with its ranges of intervals with pulsating strikes of the gong that resonate for a very long time. Intervals in perfect proportions cause a tuning in and of the body. Harmonic intervals move around, change into discords, to then again change into harmonics once more. Crystal singing bowls have a special kind of effect on emotions. Initially the child may experience an uncomfortable feeling, but soon a feeling of well-being, restfulness, and harmony takes over.[30]

Therapists can practice with simple breathing techniques with the child, such as just breathing in deeply, and then gradually breathing out again, while slightly contracting the throat so you hear a hissing sound (this is known as the calming breath). Should emotions come welling up, allow these to be here and now, let them out completely!

9. Lithophone (instrument made of Afghan black granite stone) and gong: movement with Aeolian scale

Soundscape: Melodic beat, in an Aeolian scale, with a neurosonic signal of 2 Hz (deep delta) in the background, and slow beats of a big gong. Rhythmic sounds of the stones work as a pulsating massage of the muscle tissues.
Objective: Relaxation.
Explanation: The penetrating sound of granite stone works the physical body with a sound massage, while an interference tone of 2 Hz of two low-tone stone plates puts the brain wave rhythms into deep relaxation. So this could work comfortably as a kind of daily resting cure; you can set a time to do this every day so the child can look forward to it. Depending on the need, you could by all means program this track to repeat three times, in order to create a relaxation session of a good 20 minutes. This track can also be used excellently as background sound during therapy sessions.

10. Wind chimes, birds and water sounds: timeless relaxation on the waves

Soundscape: Just relaxing sounds (the sounds of water are the most relaxing nature sounds ever), several layers of wind gongs, with neurosonic effects.

Objective: The cluster frequencies of water work to purify the nervous system; the high-frequency sounds of the birds nourish the brain with energy, just like the tingling little wind chimes, which also add a kind of playfulness and carelessness, which works beneficially on depressions and negative ideations.

Explanation: A brain wave entrainment of 4 Hz has been added, on the border of theta to delta waves, causing a delicious relaxing feeling. Toward the end, the sounds become increasingly subtle. Here is a visualization you can do with this track:

Imagine sitting at the edge of a forest, looking out over a huge sandy beach, watching the waves of the sea come and go. Up high in the trees you hear the birds whistling. You are completely calm now, and you feel at peace with yourself. It is enough just to be here and now at this place, nothing more is needed. Watch the colors and the shapes, feel the sensations, be completely in the here and now. Breathe deep and let go. The length of this sound meditation is almost ten minutes.

COMBINATION AND USE OF THE TRACKS

Here follow suggestions for a specific combination of tracks to play back, for a certain occasion or effect. Many CD players have a programming feature, allowing tracks to play back uninterrupted. Of course, these are just a few possibilities, to give you an idea how this works.

"Trying out" the tracks is the most important thing a parent can do initially, in order to see how the child will react. There may be a number of different reactions; that is why it is difficult to write an exact manual how to apply these compositions. Observing, and keeping a notebook on hand to write down what is happening, is an important therapeutic part of the quest. And of course, the author and composer of this book and CD would like to hear about the findings of both parents and children.[31]

Sequence 1
Track 4—Wood
For directing attention to the sounds themselves
Track 8—Crystal singing bowls
For going within, experiencing the sound massage; possibly evoking emotional release
Track 6—Kalimba
For slowly "awaking" again, supply of happy and light energy

Sequence 2
Track 10—Wind gongs, birds, and water
For relaxing and feeling supported by the sounds, and a soft energy charge
Track 8—Crystal singing bowls
For deep relaxation of muscles and tissues; the long continuous tones cause a deep, profound tissue resonance (changing from tension to relaxation)

Sequence 3

Track 1—Tibetan singing bowls
Here the muscles are vibrated and relaxed by the multiple harmonic overtones from the singing bowls
Track 9—Lithophone (from Afghan black granite)
This tunes the body tissues, causing consciousness to turn inward.

The intensive sound from the granite stone works as a kind of acupuncture to the energy vessels (meridians) in the body. At the end of this track comes the 2 Hz neurosonic signal from two granite plates, soothing to the brain waves, and consciousness.

Sequence 4

Track 9—Lithophone; track 8—crystal singing bowls; and track 7—voice overtones
This sequence of sounds is deliciously relaxing and soothing. It can also be listened to before going to sleep.

Sequence 5

Track 4—Wood, followed by track 10—Wind chimes, birds, and water
This helps one move from waking consciousness toward a "snoozel space" within.

Sequence 6

Track 6—Kalimba
This track create a relaxing atmosphere, for instance, to wind down to get some homework done
Tracks 4 and 5—Wood, gong, marimba, and wind gong
These are effective activities, to get the energy out of the head into the body.

Sequence 7

Track 7—Overtones of the voice
Use this track as a relaxing concentration exercise.
Track 8—Crystal singing bowls and Burmese gong

This track is a great accompaniment to breathing exercises, or have the child hum along with the sounds.

Sequence 8

Track 5— Marimba
Use this to get the child moving around the room.
Track 10—Wind gongs, birds and water
Use this track to have the child relax and/or visualize while lying on the floor in between the speakers.

• • •

Maybe you can personalize your own range of tracks, depending on how your child responds to the sounds. We are eager to hear your experiences!

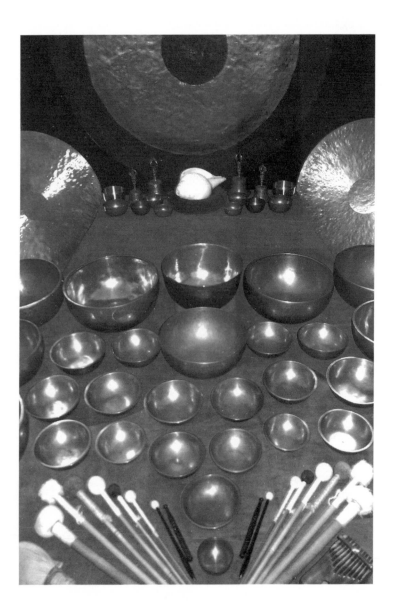

CD TIME SYNOPSIS

1. Tibetan singing bowls: acoustical neurosonic signal (gong) and rhythmic movement 8:10
2. Chinese wind chime and Burmese gong: timeless movements 7:00
3. Cymbals and Chinese gong: experiencing extreme frequencies 5:20
4. Wooden xylophone and Burmese gong: experiencing rest and movement 6:35
5. Marimba and wind chime: mobile and restful 5:10
6. Kalimba, Chinese gong and Tibetan singing bowl: relaxing into the pentatonic 5:45
7. Voice and overtones: searching for and discovering the hidden sounds behind the voice 9:40
8. Crystal singing bowls and Burmese gong 8:00
9. Lithophone and gong: movement with Aeolian scale 7:20
10. Wind chimes, birds, and water sounds: timeless relaxation on the waves 9:45

Total playing time: 72:46 minutes

RECOMMENDED MUSIC

There are many examples of classical and new age music and neurosonic sounds that can be used in coaching an ADHD child. This use can be very direct, in coherence with one or more therapies, but it can also be applied in the living room or nursery as a general background. Perhaps you already have your own preferences; or you can get some advice in your local new age store.

Classical
It has been demonstrated that the somewhat slower kinds (*adagio* or *largo*) of movements from the Baroque period can work very favorably. This music is mainly soothing, but it gives also a feeling of optimism and clarity because of the rather constant rhythm of (about) one count per second, together with the general character, which is mostly light, cheerful, and delicate. Some examples are: Adagio from Concerto Grosso, opus 6 no. 8 (Corelli); Largo from Viola d'amore Concerto in d (Vivaldi); Poco adagio from the Fourth Symphony (Mahler); Largo from the Oboe Concerto in b (Vivaldi); Allegro from the Oboe Quartet in f, KV370 (Mozart); Allegro assai from the Violin Concerto nr 2 (Bach).

New Age Music
While making selections of this music try to have a preference for acoustical instruments, because these are recognizable to the children. Still, we do not need to exclude electronic instruments; certainly when the sound is with acoustical ones. In this kind of music there is often a combination with nature sounds. This may stimulate the child's fantasy—with eyes closed—enormously, with or without an accompanying story. There are just too many examples to mention here. New age shops have big selections, and their staff can help you choose. Very popular still is the uncomplicated music of Mike Rowland, for instance his first and best, *The Fairy Ring*. Well-known other names are: Aeoliah, Joel Andrews, Erik Berglund, Deuter, Steven Halpern, Jim Oliver, and Pushkar—just to name a few.

Neurosonic sounds

Neurosonic sounds should be applied very specifically and administered mostly within the process of a therapy. Others can be used at home. For instance, there are specific recordings that can be used simply to doze off more easily into a deep sleep. It is recommended to always listen to these sounds through headphones, with attention to what is right and left. As an alternative, the child can also sit or lie down in between two big loudspeakers.

Some pleasant and effective examples are Ultra Meditation® (vols. 1, 2, 3, and 6) and Kelly Howell's Brain Sync® series. Also the 4-CD box Brainwave Suite® from Jeffrey Thompson is excellent. The Monroe recordings (HemiSync®) are effective, but personally I find these not fit this specific use, because their sound structures are too somber.[32]

NOTES

1. According to the Dutch association Balans, an co-ordinating address for ADHD and ADD.
2. Similar criteria are to be found with every authority concerned with the subject. These are enumerated at their web sites and used by physicians, therapists, and teachers. For example, the American Academy of Pediatrics' guidelines is available at http://aappolicy.aappublications.org/cgi/reprint/pediatrics;105/5/1158.pdf (*Pediatrics* 105, no. 5 [May 2000]:1158).
3. In his book *ADHD, probleem of uitdaging* (available only in Dutch).
4. In her excellent book *Understanding Your Life through Color* (Carlsbad, CA: Starling Publishers, 1986).
5. Find out more about fluoride at www.fluoridealert.org.
6. Detailed information is found in Sam Ziff, *Silver Dental Fillings: The Toxic Time Bomb* (Santa Fe, NM: Aurora Press, 1984) and Sherry A. Rogers, *Tired or Toxic: A Blueprint for Health* (Vineland, NJ: Prestige Publications, 1990) and on Dr. Joseph Mercola's web site (www.mercola.com).
7. See the many articles by Dr. Mark Sircus, O.M.D., Director International Medical Veritas Association, www.imva.info.
8. *Idem*, web site of Dr. Mark Sircus.
9. There are many good books on the subject of meal preparation and sharing, for instance, Donald Ardell, *14 Days to Wellness: The Easy, Effective, and Fun Way to Optimum Health* (Novato, CA: New World Library, 1999).
10. Watch for quality when choosing a supplement! Many vitamin and mineral supplements are ineffective if used or combined incorrectly. A naturopath can help you put together a supplement regimen. Lots of people do it, but it actually can be unsafe to take supplements on your own without know-how. Just because it's a seemingly innocent herb, mineral, or vitamin, and not a prescription drug,

doesn't mean it can do no harm! Of course there are good exceptions, like Synaptol®, Focus®, Ocean Minerals® and ConcenTrace® (see chapter 5), which are tested blends that have been in circulation a long time. Global Light Network (www.globallight.net) is a good source of information about supplements.

11. Read for instance Dharma Singh Khalsa, MD., *Food as Medicine: How to Use Diet, Vitamins, Juices and Herbs for a Healthier, Happier and Longer Life* (New York: Atria Books, 2003), Rudolph Ballentine, MD, *Diet & Nutrition*) Himalayan International Institute, 1987).

12. See also www.milksucks.com.

13. William Dufty's book *Sugar Blues* (New York: Warner Books, 1986)) was in the1970's a real eye opener for many sugar addicts. Many books about the subject have followed; many studies confirmed his view: sugar is detrimental to your health.

14. Read Karen Y. Mileson *Our Energetic Evolution in Healing: Free Yourself From the Unseen Forces That Can Make You Sick* (Steamboat Springs, CO: Energetics Research Publishing, 2006). For example, in March 2007, the French Ministry of Health sent out a warning regarding mobile phone usage: see www.nextup.org/pdf/MinistereSanteDepliantExtTelephoneMobileSanteEtSecuriteDiffusionNextupFrance.pdf.

15. The use of Ritalin is increasing at a frightening speed. See also Chapter 5.

16. Source: Dutch bureau of statistics. Children in Great Britain receive the equivalent of more than four doses of hyperactivity drugs every year, a study showed in March 2007. The use of drugs to treat hyperactivity in children has almost trebled worldwide since 1993, according to US researchers. Figures showed that spending on medication for ADHD in the UK rose 31 percent from £ 12.4 million between 1999 and 2003. (Source: *Weekly Telegraph*, March 2007).

17. According to a research in a thesis from Adrianne Faber, University of Groningen, September 19th, 2006.

18. You can read Dr. Peter R. Breggin's testimony before the U.S. House of Representatives Subcommittee on Oversight and Investigations Committee on Education and the Workforce on the harmful side effects of these drugs at www.breggin.com/classaction.html. Dr. Breggin was Director of the International Center for the Study of Psychiatry and Psychology when he testified September 29, 2000.
19. The majority of medicine for children does not comply with official protocol. Up to now, medical attendants assumed that the effects of medicines were more or less the same in children compared to adults, but often this is not the case. Not only are children smaller in size, they also have different metabolism. Much more research is needed. You will find very clear and effective guidelines at http://www.maximizeyourmetabolism.com.
20. Tijn Touber, "Mending Minds" in *Ode* 6 (August, 2003). Available online at www.odemagazine.com.
21. Many thanks to Lisa Borstlap; for more information visit www.genezendtekenen.nl
22. For example, a fairly well-absorbed preparation for ADHD children is ConcenTrace® (in tablets or fluid), or Elemental Magnesium® (was earlier Complete Magnesium®). More info: www.vitals.nl.
23. Masaru Emoto, *The Hidden Messages in Water*
24. You can see his amazing pictures of water crystals at: www.collectivewisdominitiative.org/vibration2.htm.
25. For instance on tracks 4, 6, and 8 of the CD.
26. In the hospital they use EEG-scans for neurological measurements; there is also more simple equipment you can use at home.
27. Ingo Steinbach, *Klangtherapie* (not published in English), and Joachim-Ernst Berendt, *The Third Ear: On Listening to the World* (New York: Henry Holt & Co, 1992).
28. I use this extensively with my own *Relaxperience* CD series, to make the relaxation much more effective and complete.
29. You can read more about singing bowls' effects in my book

and CD package, *The Unique Singing Bowl*, and *Singing Bowls* by Eva Rudy Jansen and Dick de Ruiter.

30. You can find a comprehensive description about crystal singing bowl sounds in my book and CD package, *Crystal & Sound.*

31. You may write to us in care of the publisher.

32. Available via mail order from Tools for Exploration, www.toolsforexploration.com.

RESOURCES

We hope that the following lists of web sites, books, and organizations will help you on your search for help coping with your or your child's ADHD.

Web Sites: General Information

About ADHD – A Fact Sheet by Dr. Barkley: www.russell-barkley.org/adhd-facts.htm

ADHD and Giftedness (About.com article): http://add.about.com/cs/education/a/gifted.htm
Siblings and ADHD: (About.com article): www.add.about.com/od/parentingchildrenwithadd/a/siblings2.htm

Adult ADHD online self-test: www.psychcentral.com/addquiz.htm

ADHD Support Groups in Australia: www.adders.org/ausmap.htm

Australian Government Health Insite web page with links to health services: healthinsite.gov.au/topics/Health_Services.

Eli Lilly and Co (a pharmaceutical company) web site with helpful information about diagnosing, treating, and living with ADHD: www.adhd.com

International Medical Veritas Association site directed by Mark Allen Sircus Ac., OMD: www.imva.info

Understanding ADHD: www.understandingadhd.com, a collaboration with Healthology (www.healthology.com), 500 7th Ave, 14th Fl, New York, NY 10018

Web Sites: Healing Techniques

Simon Heather's "The Healing Power of Sound" article: www.positivehealth.com/permit/Articles/Sound_and_Music/heather64.htm

Web Sites: Nutrition

International site about what you need to know about food, supplements, additives: www.food-info.net
World's Healthiest Foods, a service of the non-profit George Mateljan Foundation for nutrition information about all healthy foods: www.whfoods.com

READ MORE

Amen, Daniel. *Healing ADD: The Breakthrough Program That Allows You to See and Heal the 6 Types of ADD.* New York: Berkley, 2001.

American Psychiatric Association. *Diagnostic and Statistical Manual of Mental Disorders*, Fourth Edition, Text Revision. Washington, DC: American Psychiatric Association, 2000.

Ardell, Donald. *14 Days to Wellness: The Easy, Effective, and Fun Way to Optimum Health.* Novato, CA: New World Library, 1999.

Barkley, Russell A. *Attention-Deficit Hyperactivity Disorder: A Handbook for Diagnosis and Treatment.* New York: Guilford Press, 1998.

———. *A New Look at ADHD: Inhibition, Time, and Self-Control* (DVD with manual). New York: Guilford Press, 2006.

———. *Taking Charge of ADHD: The Complete, Authoritative Guide for Parents.* Revised edition. New York: Guilford Press, 2000.

Block, Mary Ann. *No More Ritalin: Treating ADHD without Drugs.* New York: Kensington, 2006.

Campbell, Don. *The Mozart Effect: Tapping the Power of Music to Heal the Body, Strengthen the Mind, and Unlock the Creative Spirit.* New York: HarperCollins, 2001.

———. *The Mozart Effect for Children: Awakening Your Child's Mind, Health and Creativity with Music.* New York: HarperCollins, 2002.

Carroll, Lee and Jan Tober. *The Indigo Children: The New Kids Have Arrived.* Carlsbad, CA: Hay House, 1999.

Dewhurst-Maddock, Olivea. *The Book of Sound Therapy.* London: Gaia Books, 2000.

Fellman, Wilma F. *The Other Me: Poetic Thoughts on ADD for Adults, Kids and Parents.* Plantation, FL: Specialty Press, 1997.

Fenichel, Gerald M. *Clinical Pediatric Neurology.* Philadelphia: W. B. Saunders, 2001.

Gordon, Michael. *ADHD-Hyperactivity: A Consumer's Guide.* Dewitt, NY: GSI Publications, 1991.

Hartmann, Thom. *Thom Hartmann's Complete Guide to ADHD: Help for Your Family at Home, School and Work.* Nevada City, CA: Underwood Books, 2000.

Hallowell, Edward M., and John J. Ratey. *Driven to Distraction.* New York: Touchstone, 1995.

Joudry, Rafaele. *Why Aren't I Learning?* Sound Therapy International, 2004.

Joudry, Patricia and Rafaele. *Sound Therapy: Music to Recharge Your Brain.* Gerringong, NSW: Sound Therapy International, 1999.

Lark, Liz. *Yoga for Kids.* Toronto: Firefly Books, 2003.

Leeds, Joshua. *The Power of Sound: How to Manage Your Personal Soundscape for a Vital, Productive, and Healthy Life.* Includes a CD. Rochester, VT: Healing Arts Press, 2001.

The PDR Family Guide to Natural Medicines & Healing Therapies. New York: Ballantine, 2000.

Reif, Sandra. *The ADD/ADHD Checklist: An Easy Reference for Parents & Teachers.* Hoboken, NJ: Jossey-Bass, 1997.

Sircus, Mark. *Heart Health.* IMVA Publications, e-book available at www.imva.info.

———. *Transdermal Magnesium Therapy.* Chandler, AZ: Phaelos Books & Mediawerks, 2006.

Solanto, Mary V., Arnsten, Amy F. T., and Castellanos, Xavier. *Stimulant Drugs and ADHD, Basic and Clinical Neuroscience.* New York: Oxford University Press, 2001.

Tappe, Nancy Ann. *Understanding Your Life through Color.* Carlsbad, CA: Starling Pubishers, 1986.

Teeter, Phyllis Anne. *Interventions for ADHD.* New York: Guilford Press, 1998.

Weingartner, Paul L. *ADHD Handbook for Families: A Guide to Communicating with Professionals.* Washington, DC: Child & Family Press, 1999.

Wender, Paul H. *ADHD: Attention Deficit Hyperactivity Disorder in Children and Adults.* New York: Oxford University Press, 2000.

Useful Addresses

In the United States

Association of Waldorf Schools of North America
337 Oak Grove St
Minneapolis MN 5540
Phone (612) 870-8310; fax (612) 870-8316
awsna@awsna.org
www.awsna.org

Montessori Foundation
The International Montessori Council
2400 Miguel Bay Dr
PO Box 130
Terra Ceia Island, FL 34250-0130
(941) 729-9565 (941) 729-9594
www.montessori.org

National Institute of Mental Health
Public Information and Communications Branch
601 Executive Blvd Rm 8184 MSC 9663
Bethesda, MD 20893-0663
Phone (in U.S.): 1 866 615 6464 (toll free), 301-443-4513 (local)
Fax: 301 443 4279
E-mail: nimhinfo@nih.gov
www.nimh.nih.gov; For a guide to local services, go to
http://www.nimh.nih.gov/healthinformation/gettinghelp.cfm

In Great Britain

Adders
45 Vincent Close
Broadstairs
Kent CT10 2ND
England
Phone (in UK): 870 950 3693
E-mail: support@adders.org
www.adders.org

ADDISS
PO Box 340
Edgware
Middlesex HA8 9HL
Phone (in UK): 0208 906 9068
Fax: 0208 959 0727
E-mail: info@addiss.co.uk
www.addiss.co.uk

ADHD UK Alliance
209-211 City Road
London EC1V 1JN
Phone (in UK): 0207 608 8760
Fax: 0208 770 1554
E-mail: info@adhdalliance.org.uk
www.adhdalliance.org.uk

Parentline Plus
520 Highgate Studios
53-79 Highgate Rd
London NW5 1TL
Phone (in UK): 0808 800 2222
E-mail: contact@parentlineplus.org.uk
www.parentlineplus.org.uk

The Steiner Waldorf Schools Fellowship
Kidbrooke Park
Forest Row
East Sussex RH18 5JA
Phone (in UK): 01342 822115
Fax: 01342 826004
E-mail@swsf.org.uk
www.steinerwaldorf.org.uk

In Australia

Behavioural Neuropathy Clinic
Jacques Duff, Director
2/314 Manningham Rd
Doncaster, VIC 3108
Phone (in Australia): 9848 9100
Fax: 9848 9300
www.adhd.com.au

Canberra & Queanbeyan ADD Support Group, Inc.
PO Box 717, Mawson, ACT 2607
Phone (in Australia): 02 62901984, Fax: 02 62864475
E-mail: addact@shout.org.au

Sound Therapy International
Commercial Unit 2
9 Bergin St
Gerringong, NSW 2534
Phone in Australia: 130 055 7796; international: 61 2 42344534;
USA: 1 800 323 9956
Fax: +61 (0)2 42344537
E-mail: info@soundtherapyinternational.com
www.soundtherapyinternational.com

About the Author and the Musician

DICK DE RUITER (1951) has been a yoga teacher and dietician since 1969, and has specialized since 1980 in the harmonious possibilities of sound. In the 1970s, he introduced new age music to his home country, the Netherlands, with his mail order business Sono Music of Silence. Later he specialized in neurosonic sounds and effects with his Odyssey series. He has offered numerous workshops about the effects of sound and special music in daily life. He has his own series of narrated relaxation and visualization, the Relaxperience® CDs. He writes and translates books on yoga, sound, and related subjects. Today, he lives and works in the south of France. Readers can learn more about his work at www.maisondesmiracles.nl.

DANNY BECHER (1953) has been a musician since his twenties, and studied Eastern classical music and singing while living in India for eight years. Since 1981 he has been living and working in the Netherlands as a gifted singer, musician, and teacher. He holds a degree in Western classical music and is also a qualified choirmaster. He has performed in concerts in many countries with singing bowls and overtone singing, and is a member of the Swedish TONUS-ensemble. Find out more at www.danny-becher.com.